CLEAN LIVING
EAT CLEAN
ALL YEAR

Join Luke and Scott on the CLEAN LIVING journey

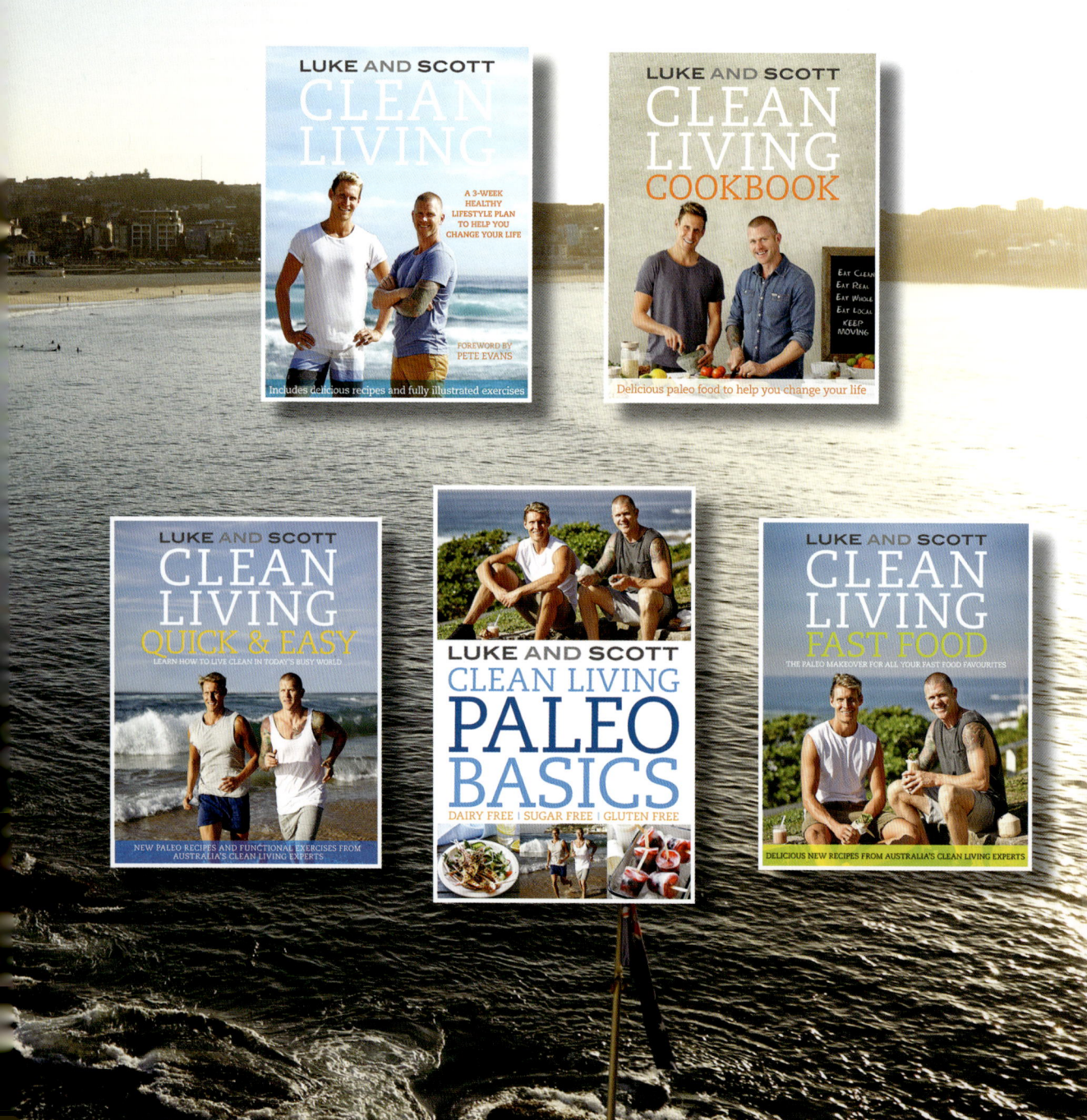

LUKE HINES AND SCOTT GOODING

CLEAN LIVING

EAT CLEAN ALL YEAR

OVER 70 OF YOUR FAMILY FAVOURITES GIVEN THE PALEO MAKEOVER

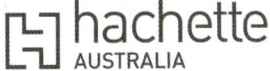
hachette
AUSTRALIA

hachette
AUSTRALIA

Published in Australia and New Zealand in 2015
by Hachette Australia
(an imprint of Hachette Australia Pty Limited)
Level 17, 207 Kent Street, Sydney NSW 2000
www.hachette.com.au

10 9 8 7 6 5 4 3 2 1

National Library of Australia
Cataloguing-in-Publication data:

Hines, Luke, author.
Eat clean all year/Luke Hines, Scott Gooding.

978 0 7336 3384 3 (paperback)

Cooking.
Nutrition.
Cooking (Natural foods).
Well-being.

Other Creators/Contributors: Gooding, Scott, author.

641.563

Cover design and text design by Liz Seymour
Typeset in PMN Caecilia by Agave Creative
Photography by Steve Brown
Food preparation by Tracey Meharg
Styling by Trish Heagerty
Props provided by Studio Enti (www.studioenti.com.au), and
   Pulp Creative Paper (www.pulpcreativepaper.com.au)
Printed in China by Toppan Leefung Printing Limited

Contents

Introduction   vi

A Note on Ingredients   ix

The Warmer Months   1

The Cooler Months   59

Year-Round Essentials   113

Index   144

Introduction

Hi guys, can you believe it? Here we are again with our sixth book in the Clean Living series. It has been absolutely incredible sharing our passion for a healthy lifestyle with you. Throughout this awesome health and wellness journey we're all on together, we have done our best to empower you with the skills to live your best life. In our earlier books, we introduced you to the most nutrient-dense foods on the planet and taught you to move your body in a way that is both functional and fun. Now we want to help you embrace the Clean Living lifestyle all year round, which is why you have this book in your hot little hands.

It's easy to eat clean in summer, when all you want is something light and fresh, and you're baring all down at the beach, but with the right recipes you can eat clean no matter what the season, experiencing all the year has to offer – including the rich, heartwarming dishes we all love in the colder months. Eating clean shouldn't get in the way of a good time, either, and with countless celebrations throughout the year such as Easter, Christmas and birthdays, we want you to have your cake and eat it too!

Too often we hear people say that to be healthy you have to deny yourself the foods and flavours you love. Well, we cannot disagree more. We believe that healthy food is actually the most delicious food out there, because it is real produce, prepared in the most ethical and loving way, and with flavours that complement it, without trying to turn it into something it is not. Simplicity is key with clean food, guys – let the produce speak for itself and allow its natural flavour to be the hero of the dish.

Our Clean Living makeovers on these seasonal favourites are so good that our recipes are more delicious than the originals. Compare a birthday cake full of processed sugars and artificial colours with a nutrient-dense wholefood cake made with antioxidant-rich cacao and energy-boosting coconut oil. You know which one would taste better – and you'd look and feel better after eating it, too. We are so incredibly confident about our flavour combinations that we give you this guarantee: if you serve up one of our recipes to your friends and family, they won't even know they're eating 'healthy'. Our food is just good, honest home cooking at its finest, without anything fake, artificial or refined.

It's important to us that our recipes are quick to prepare and good value for money, too, whether you're cooking for one or a whole family. The less time you spend in the kitchen, the more time you can spend with loved ones – that's what life is about, spending time with those we care about, and doing that over shared food is even better. The joy and comfort we get from eating good food shouldn't come at an exorbitant cost, so we keep recipe ingredients to a minimum while also choosing fresh produce, cuts of meat and pantry staples that are affordable.

We believe our sustainable and practical philosophy on food and nutrition will help you live your best life. Why? Well, how we fuel our body has a direct result on how we look and feel. And if we put in the best, most nutrient-dense foods on the planet, while avoiding those that cause us harm, we are giving our bodies the best chance to thrive in every single way.

Be clear, be present and be excited to tackle each and every one of these recipes with love, share them with your friends and family, and, most of all, remember to eat clean, all year round.

Luke & Scott xx

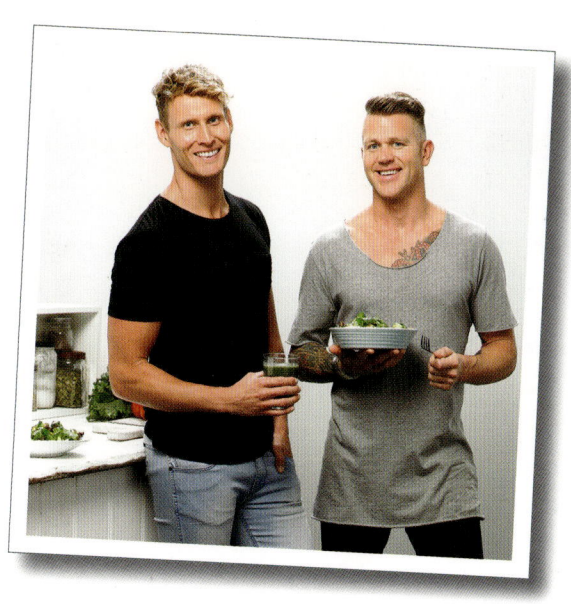

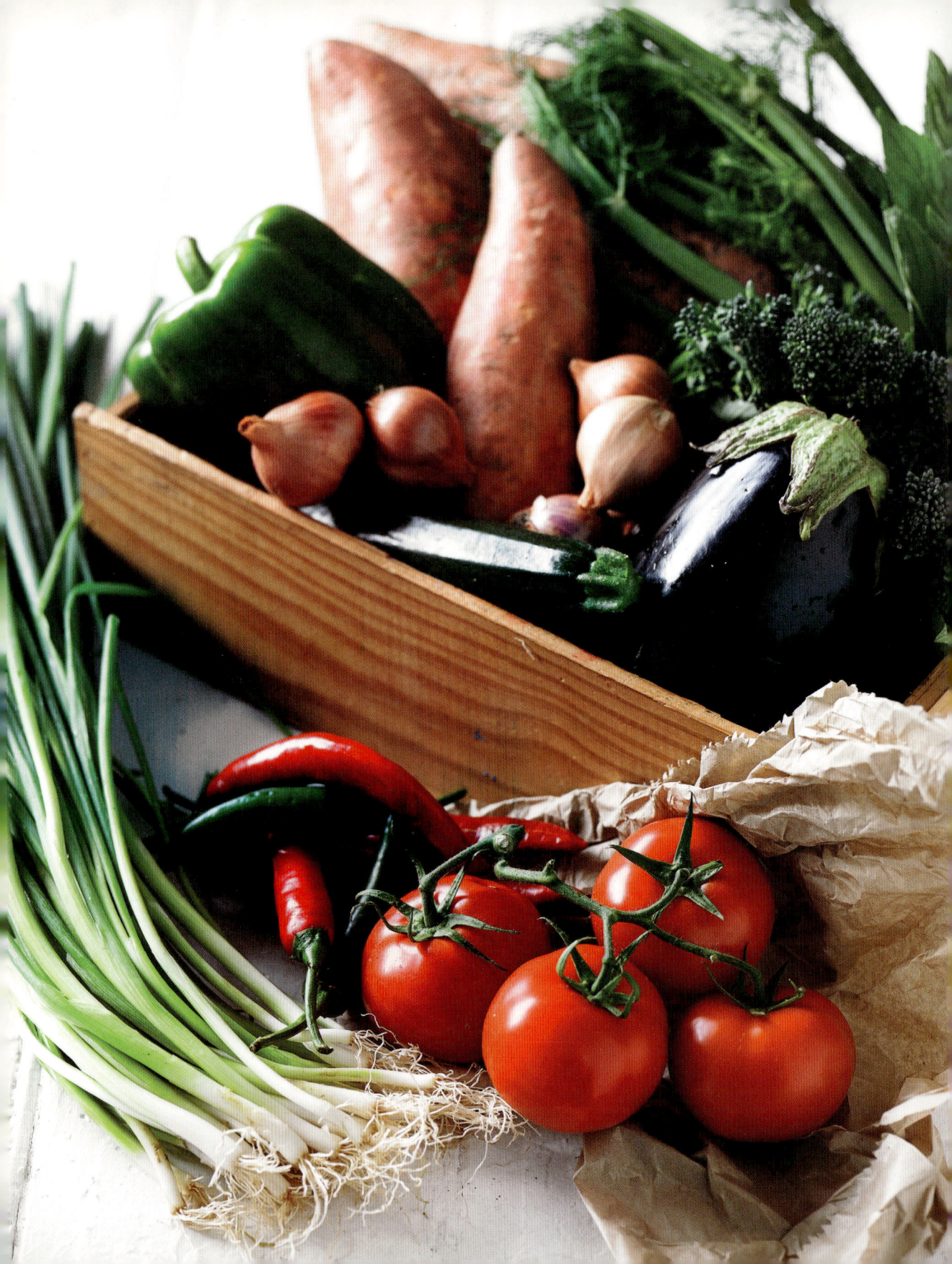

A Note on Ingredients

We know that the quality of energy you get out of your body is only as good as the quality of food you put into it. We always try to use the best ingredients we can, which usually means organic, biodynamic and free-range. We also like to support local businesses supplying sustainable, ethically produced foods.

When you look at the ingredients in our recipes, always bear in mind that:

- Eggs are biodynamic and free-range, and chicken is organic and free-range.

- Pork is organic, and bacon is nitrate-free.

- Beef and lamb are grass-fed.

- Fish are sustainably caught or farmed, wherever possible.

- Fruit and veggies are fresh, as are garlic, ginger and herbs, unless otherwise noted.

- Dates are always fresh and organic. We like the soft, fat, juicy kind.

- Citrus juices are always freshly squeezed, not bottled.

- We often use coconut oil for frying, but you can substitute lard, tallow, duck fat, bacon fat, butter or ghee.

- Coconut oil and coconut cream, milk and water are all organic.

- Olive oil is always extra-virgin.

- Apple cider vinegar is raw.

- Honey and maple syrup are pure and organic.

- Coffee and tea are organic and fair-trade.

- We use organic sea salt, and black pepper is always freshly ground.

- We also use non-stick baking paper and aluminium-free baking powder and bicarb soda!

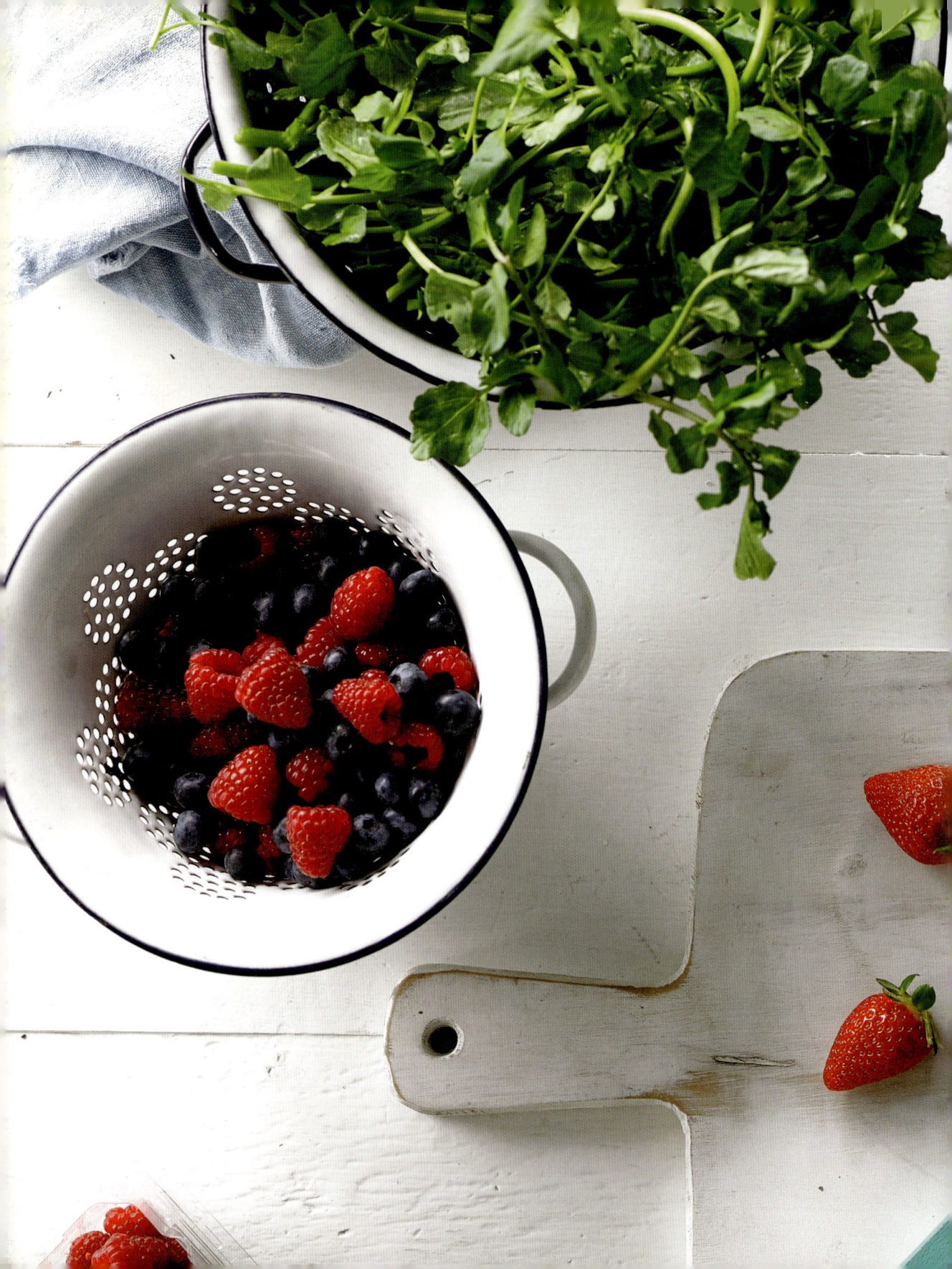

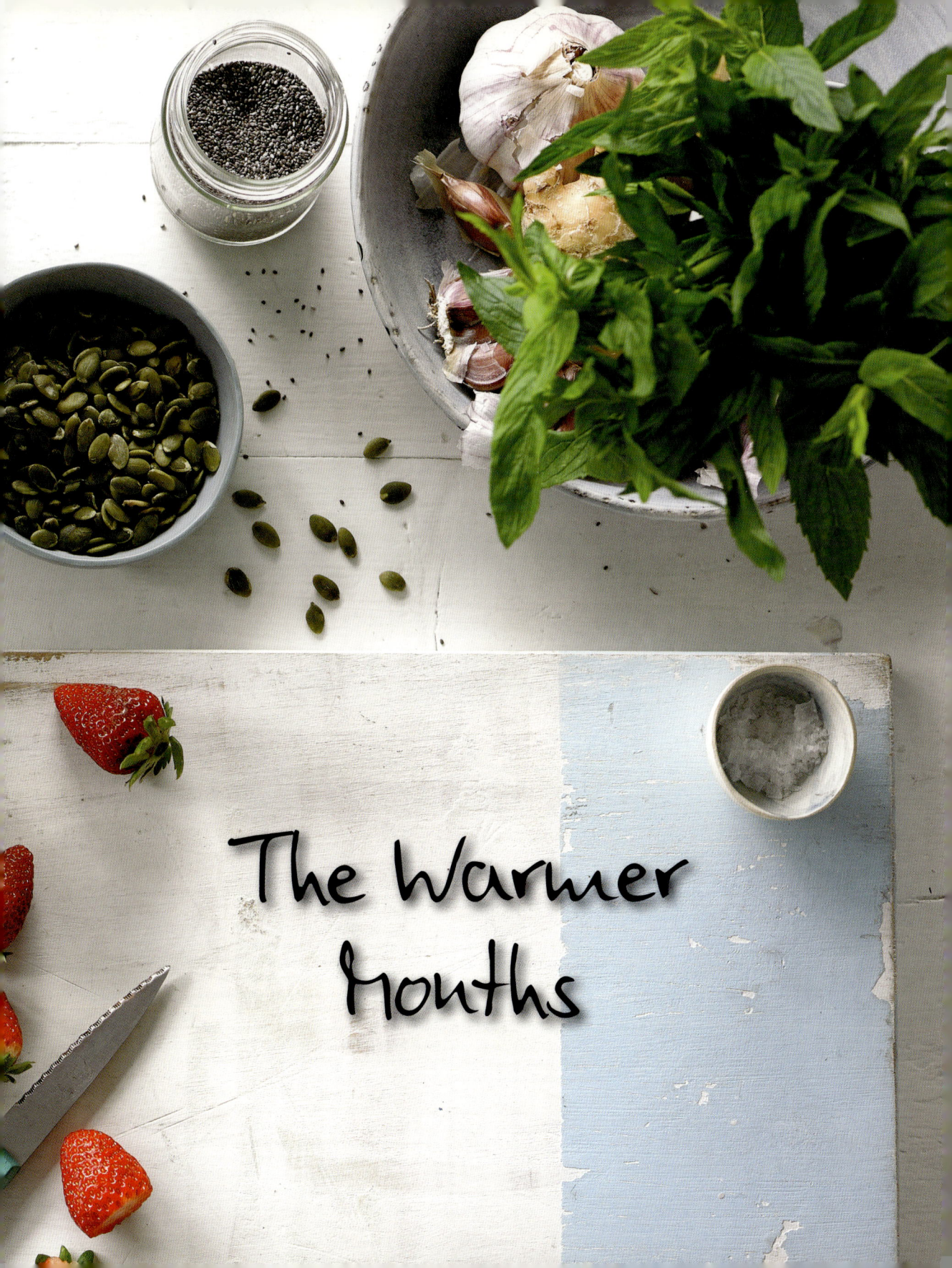

The Warmer Months

Whole Snapper with Fennel and Pistachio Crust   5

Party Frittata   6

Crispy Chilli Chicken   9

Prawn Salad with Nuoc Cham   10

Sweet Potato and Crab Croquettes   13

Cauliflower Korma Curry   14

Burgers or Meatballs   17

Crispy Skin Barramundi with Pico de Gallo   18

Christmas Turkey with Chorizo Stuffing   21

Garlic and Rosemary Focaccia   22

Mini Meatloaves with Avo Smash   24

Kiwi Marinated Skirt Steak   27

Crispy Fish Tacos with Guacamole   28

Luke and Scott's Pâté   31

Tea-Smoked Trout Blini   32

Icy Poles   35

Mango Lime Chia Pudding   36

Lime Mousse with Toasted Nut Crumble   39

Salted Caramel Choc Fudge   40

Coconut and Mango Semifreddo   43

Red Velvet Celebration Cake   44

Neapolitan Ice-Cream Cake   47

Christmas Pudding with Spiced Cream   49

Summer Trifle   51

Festive Panforte   54

Individual Christmas Cakes   57

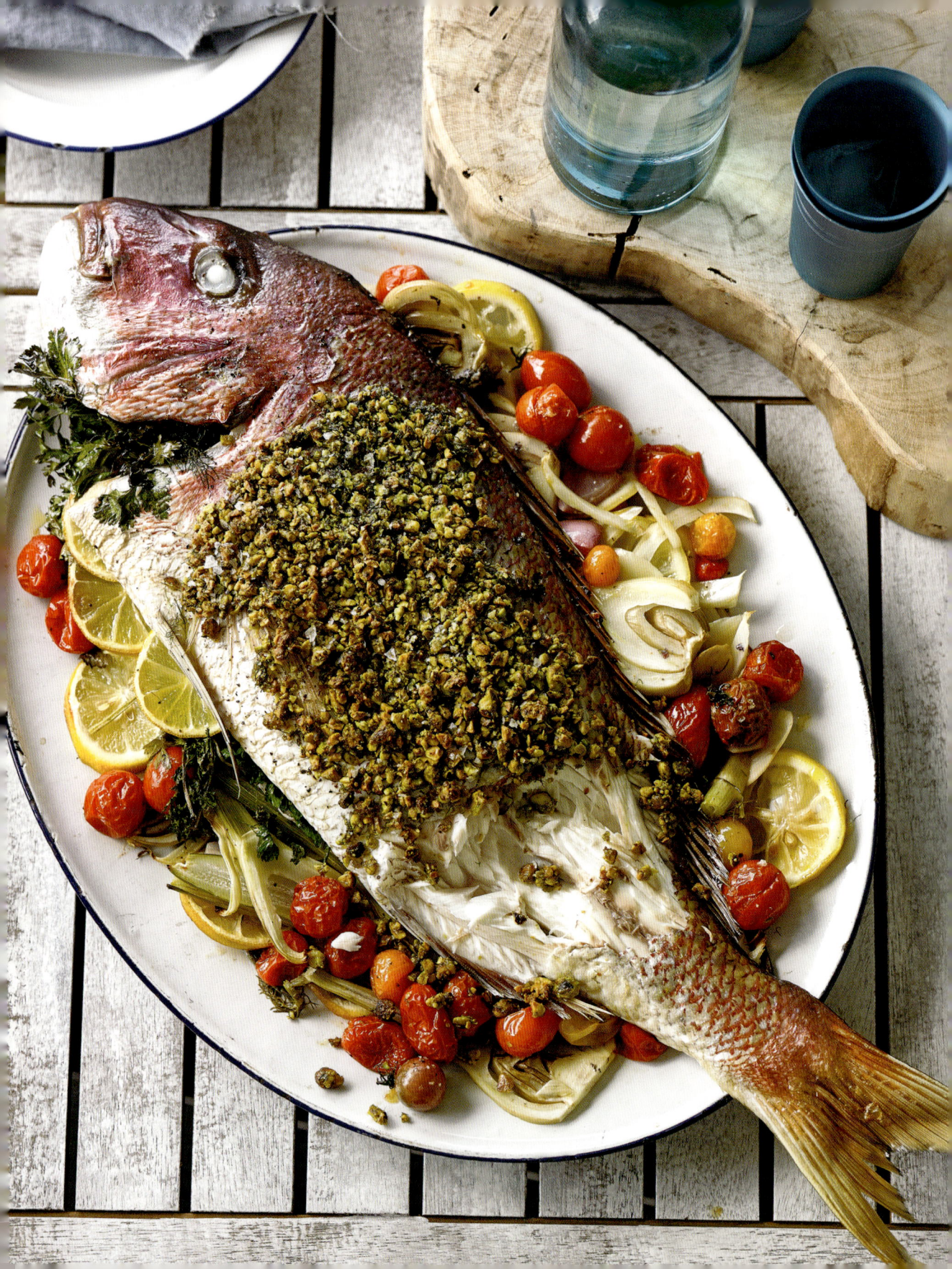

Whole Snapper with Fennel and Pistachio Crust

Serves 6

This recipe is a crowd fave and one we have cooked many a time. It's a perfect dish for when friends drop by or to take to a barbecue – it looks and smells amazing!

3 lemons

2 fennel bulbs, thinly sliced, with fronds removed and kept to one side

3 eschalots, roughly chopped

500 g baby heirloom tomatoes (mixed colours look good)

sea salt and ground black pepper

2.4 kg snapper, cleaned

½ bunch dill

½ bunch flat-leaf parsley

½ bunch coriander

⅓ cup pistachios

olive oil

1. Preheat your oven to 180° C and line a large baking tray with baking paper. Slice 2 of the lemons, then layer the lemon slices, fennel, eschalots and tomatoes on the tray and season with salt and pepper. Stuff the cavity of the snapper with the herbs and the remaining lemon, sliced.

2. In a food processor, blend the pistachios, fennel fronds and a dash of olive oil for 30 seconds or so, or until fairly smooth – a few bigger bits is totally fine. The mixture should hold together, but if it's too dry, drizzle in a little more olive oil and blend again.

3. Spread the mixture over the top of the fish, then put the tray in the oven for about 45 minutes, depending on the size of the fish. When the fish is cooked and the topping has baked to a hard crust, take it out of the oven. Let it rest for 5 minutes, then serve and enjoy.

Party Frittata

Serves 6

This is an awesome dish for parties. It tastes great, it's suitable for vegetarians, and it's good for you, all at the same time. It's also quick and easy to prepare, and it can cook while you're getting ready!

10 eggs

120 ml coconut cream

sea salt and ground black pepper

¼ cup coconut oil

1 red onion, sliced

2 garlic cloves, finely chopped

1 long red chilli, thinly sliced

400 g cooked mixed veggies, such as diced sweet potato, zucchini and broccoli

2 tablespoons flat-leaf parsley, chopped

1. Preheat your oven to 180°C and line a deep 28 x 36 cm baking tray with baking paper, letting the paper extend a few centimetres above the sides.
2. Crack the eggs into a bowl, then whisk in the coconut cream. Season well with salt and pepper and set the mixture aside.
3. Put the coconut oil in a large frying pan over a medium heat. When it's hot, add the onion, garlic and chilli and cook until soft and slightly golden.
4. Stir in the veggies and parsley and cook gently for 2–3 minutes, or until heated through. Season with salt and pepper, transfer to the prepared tray, then pour in the egg mixture. Put the dish in the oven and bake for 30 minutes, or until the frittata is golden on top and the egg is cooked through.
5. Leave the frittata to cool for at least 10 minutes, then cut it into portions. You can cut it in the tray or use the baking paper to lift it out in one piece and transfer it to a chopping board.

TIP: This recipe is great for using up whatever's in the fridge, so get creative and let your imagination run wild. You could try upping the protein by adding some leftover meat, like our roast lamb (see recipe on page 72). Simply swap out half the veggies for 200 grams of meat.

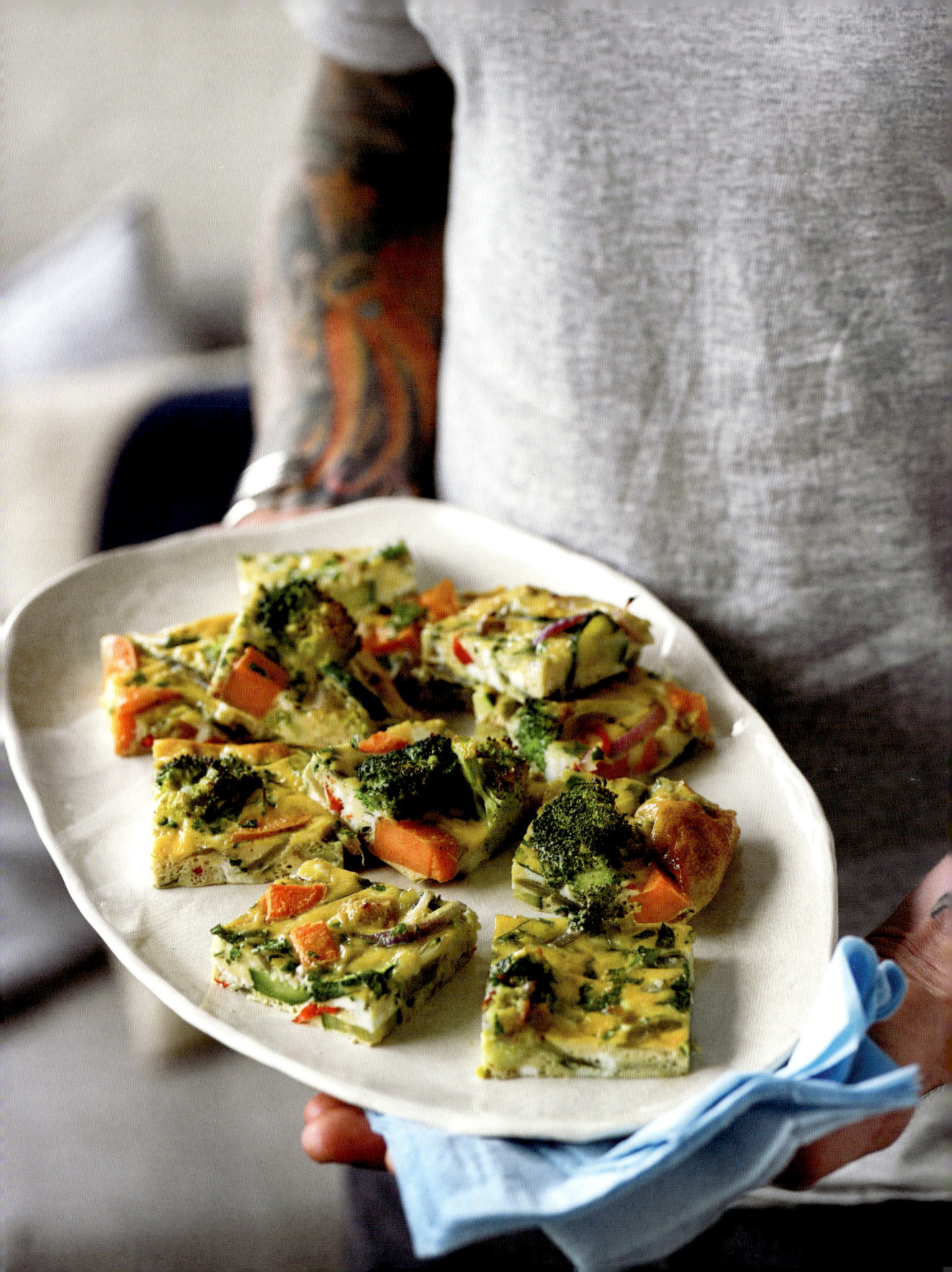

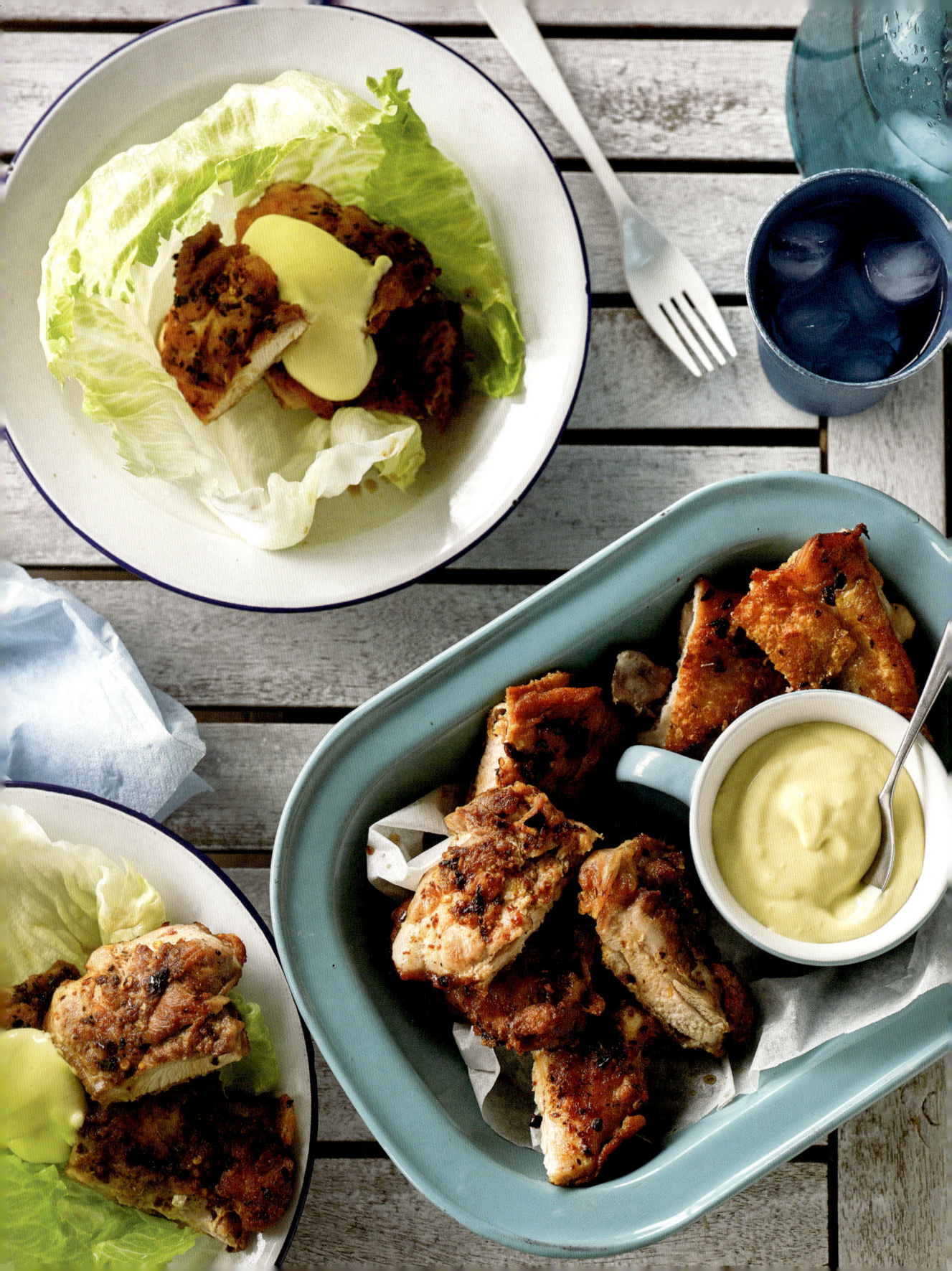

Crispy Chilli Chicken

Serves 4

The super crispy skin on these chilli chicken thighs is like pork crackling! You'll LOVE IT! Crack these little babies out at your next summer barbecue or picnic. They're definitely more-ish, so have a few extra on hand for that perfect hit of protein and good fat.

8 chicken thighs, skin on, deboned

1 tablespoon sea salt

2 teaspoons duck fat

2 teaspoons dried chilli flakes

lettuce cups, to serve

garlic aioli, to serve (see recipe on page 129)

1. Make sure the chicken thighs are super-dry by patting them down with paper towel.
2. Flatten the thighs with a meat pounder so they'll cook evenly, then season the skin with sea salt.
3. Melt the duck fat in a heavy frying pan over a medium heat and put half the chicken thighs skin side down in the hot pan. Season the meat side (not the skin side) with the dried chilli flakes.
4. Let the chicken fry, undisturbed, for 6–8 minutes, until it's crispy and golden brown. Flip it over and cook for 3 minutes, or until cooked through. Keep warm and repeat with the remaining chicken.
5. Serve with some fermented veggies or wrapped up in lettuce cups with garlic aioli.

VARIATION: Swap out the chilli for cumin and paprika for Mexican-style crispy chicken!

TIP: Try serving this with our raw cashew sour cream. Check out the recipe on page 129.

Prawn Salad with Nuoc Cham

Serves 4

This light salad is perfect on a hot night – delicious fresh prawns served with a fragrant, spicy sauce.

12 large green king prawns, peeled, de-veined, tails left on

1 teaspoon cumin seeds

1 tablespoon sesame seeds

2 teaspoons sesame oil

1 bunch Chinese broccoli, cut into 5 cm lengths

1 large red onion, cut into wedges

1 cup mint leaves

1 cup basil leaves

80 g snow pea shoot leaves

Nuoc Cham

2 tablespoons maple syrup

2 tablespoons fish sauce

2 tablespoons lime juice

1 small red chilli, finely chopped

1 small garlic clove, finely chopped

1 lemongrass stalk, trimmed, pale part only finely chopped

1. To make the nuoc cham, combine the maple syrup with ⅓ cup water in a small saucepan over a medium heat and bring to the boil. Boil for 5 minutes, or until reduced by half. Take the pan off the heat and stir through the remaining ingredients. Set the pan aside to cool.

2. To make the prawn salad, combine the prawns, cumin seeds, sesame seeds and sesame oil in a bowl. Toss together, then cover and chill for at least 1 hour.

3. Pop a large chargrill pan over a medium-high heat. When it's hot, chargrill the Chinese broccoli in batches for 1 minute each, or until just tender and lightly charred. Transfer to a serving platter. Chargrill the onion for 2–3 minutes, or until just tender and lightly charred. Transfer to the same serving platter. Add the mint, basil and snow pea shoot leaves to the platter, then toss to mix through the Chinese broccoli and onions.

4. Chargrill the prawns for 1–2 minutes, or until just cooked and lightly charred. Pop the prawns on top of the salad and spoon the nuoc cham over them. Serve warm.

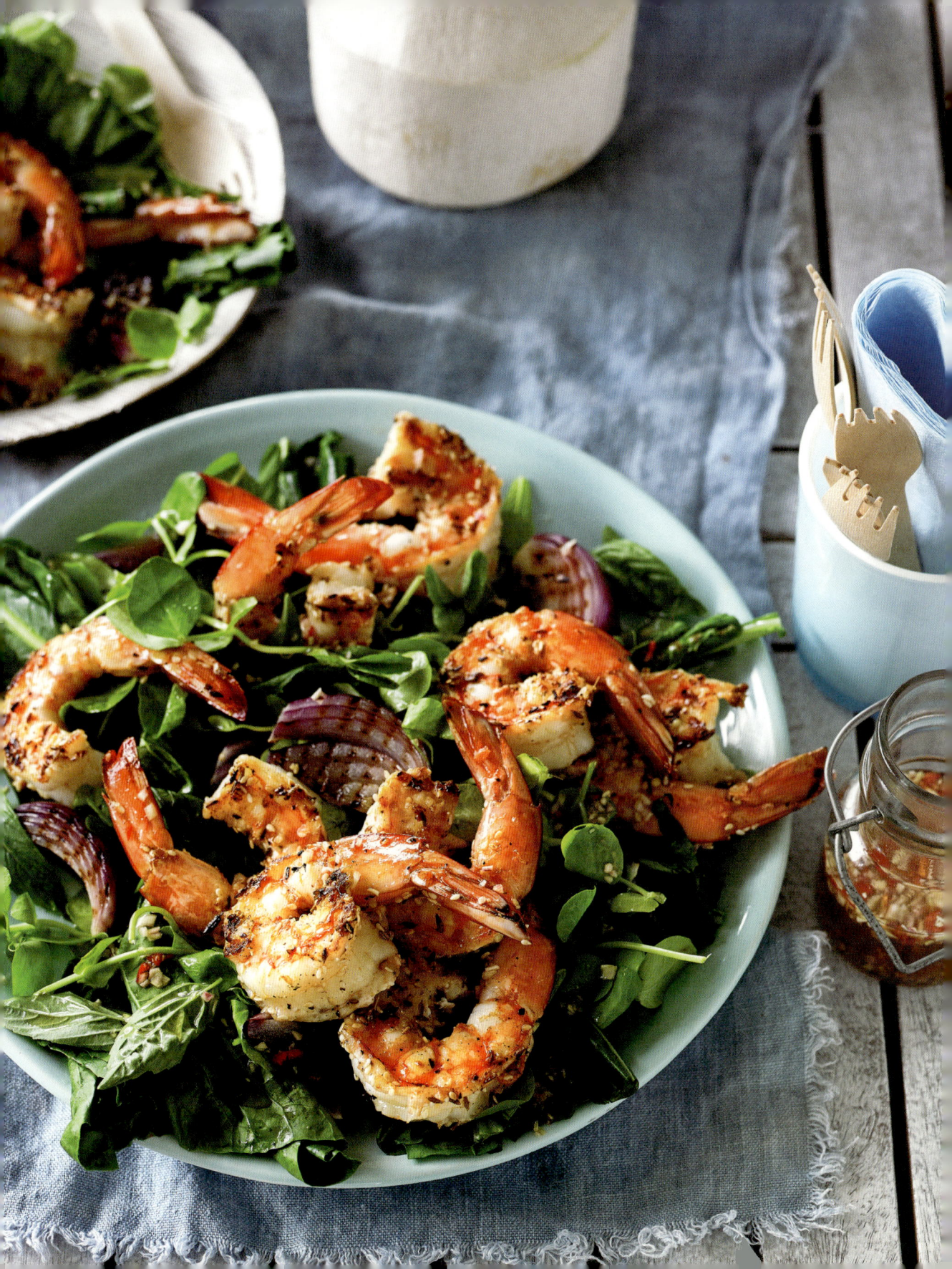

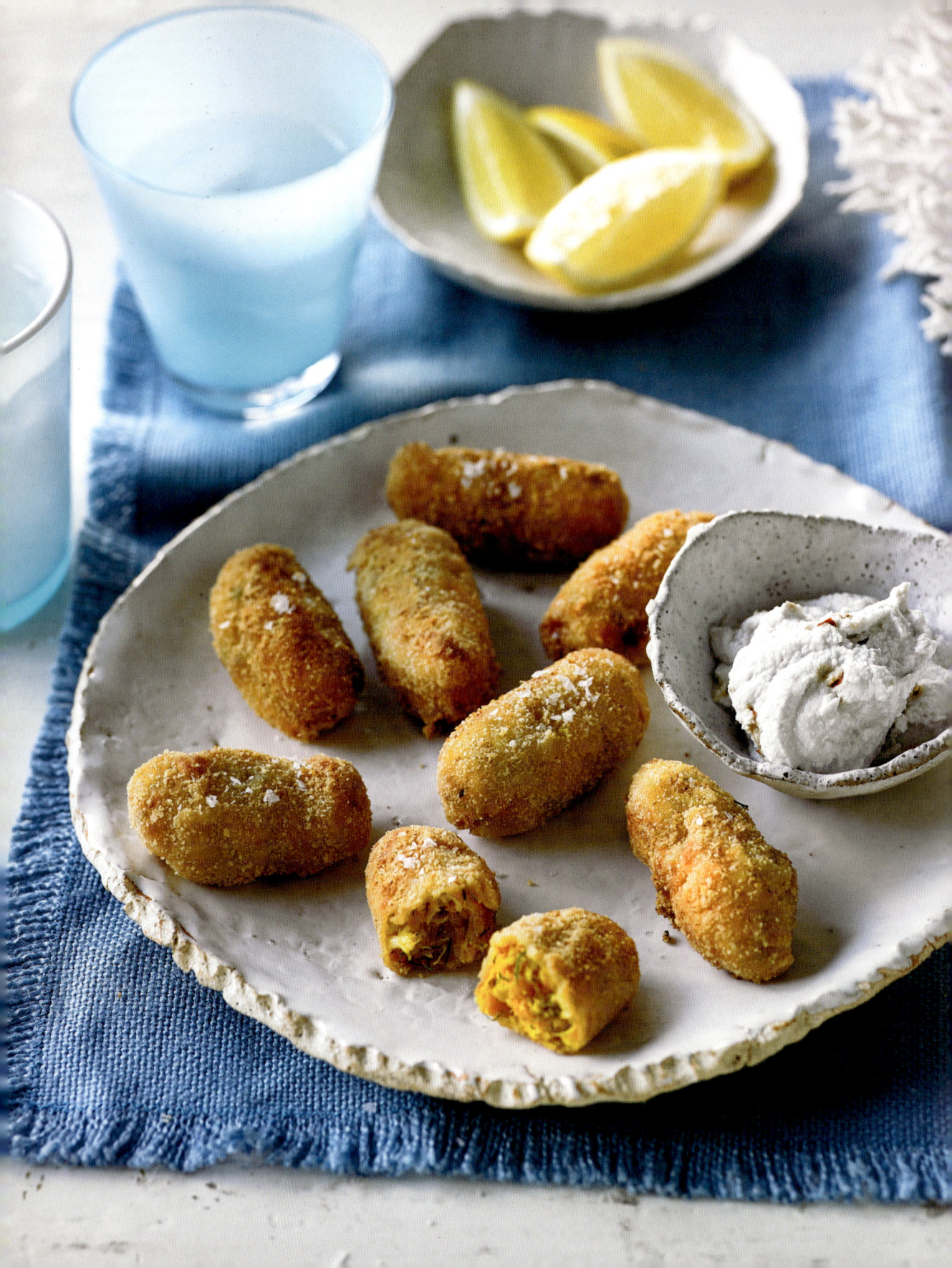

Sweet Potato and Crab Croquettes

Makes 16

When you're craving greasy fried food from your local fast-food joint, make these lightly fried healthy croquettes instead!

Croquettes

250 g peeled sweet potato, chopped

finely grated zest and juice of ½ lemon

1 egg yolk

2 tablespoons chopped dill

2 teaspoons finely grated fresh turmeric

¾ cup freshly cooked crab meat

sea salt and ground black pepper

lemon wedges, to serve

Crumb Coating

2 eggs, at room temperature

1 cup arrowroot, seasoned

2 cups almond meal, seasoned

coconut oil, for shallow-frying

Chilli Coconut Dipping Sauce

400 ml can coconut cream, chilled in fridge overnight to set

2 small red chillis, finely chopped

1 tablespoon lemon juice

1. To make the croquettes, line a baking tray with baking paper, then steam the sweet potato for 8–10 minutes, or until tender. Transfer to a heat-proof bowl and mash, then cool slightly. Add the remaining ingredients, then mix well to combine and season to taste. Take 1 tablespoon of the mixture and roll it into an oval, then put it on the baking tray. Repeat until all the mixture has been used. Cover the croquettes and chill for 1 hour.

2. To make the dipping sauce, remove the can of coconut cream from the fridge, open it and carefully scoop out the top thick layer of cream that has set firm. Combine with the chilli and lemon juice in a small bowl, then season to taste.

3. To prepare your crumb coating, whisk the eggs in a bowl with 2 tablespoons water, then set aside. Put the seasoned arrowroot in another bowl, and the seasoned almond meal in a third bowl.

4. Coat each croquette in the arrowroot, then dip it in the egg wash and roll it in the almond meal until it's evenly coated. Return the croquettes to the tray, then cover and chill for 1 hour, until they're firm and the crumb coating is set.

5. Fill a heavy saucepan with about 3 cm of coconut oil and pop it over a medium heat. When the oil is hot, shallow-fry the croquettes in batches for 3–5 minutes each. Use a slotted spoon to transfer them to paper towel to drain. Season immediately with sea salt. Serve hot with the chilli dipping sauce and lemon wedges.

Cauliflower Korma Curry

Serves 6

Paleo veggie options can be few and far between, but this is one of those recipes that tastes just as good without the meat, and the fresh produce just sings!

2 tablespoons coconut oil

1 large red onion, cut into thick
  wedges

650 g large cauliflower florets

400 ml can coconut cream

1 red capsicum, cut into
  3 cm pieces

100 g baby spinach

flaked natural almonds, toasted,
  to serve

Curry Paste

2 teaspoons cumin seeds

1 teaspoon coriander seeds

2 garlic cloves

4 cm piece ginger, peeled,
  chopped

1 teaspoon cayenne pepper

1½ teaspoons garam masala

1 overripe Roma tomato, chopped

2 tablespoons desiccated coconut

¼ cup raw almonds

1 long green chilli, chopped

1. To make the curry paste, put all of the ingredients together in a food processor. Process until smooth, adding a little water to the mixture if needed.

2. Put the coconut oil in a large saucepan over a medium heat. When it's hot, add the curry paste and cook, stirring, for 3 minutes, or until fragrant.

3. Add the onion and cauliflower and cook, stirring occasionally, for 5 minutes, or until the onion is just starting to soften. Add the coconut cream and bring to the boil, then turn the heat down to low. Simmer, covered, for 10 minutes. Stir in the capsicum and simmer for 2 minutes more, or until the cauliflower is just tender.

4. Take the pan off the heat and stir in the spinach until it wilts. Season to taste before serving.

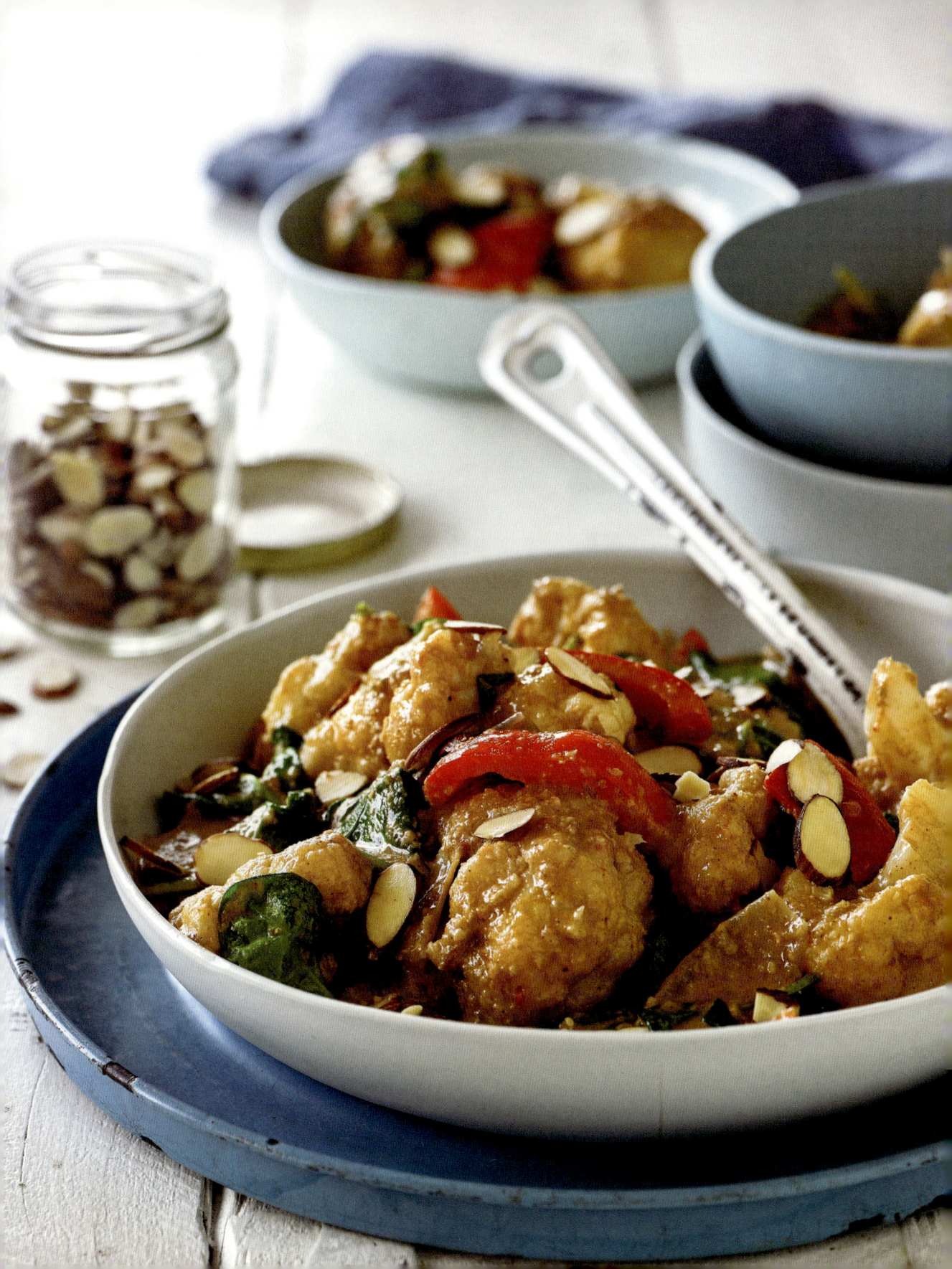

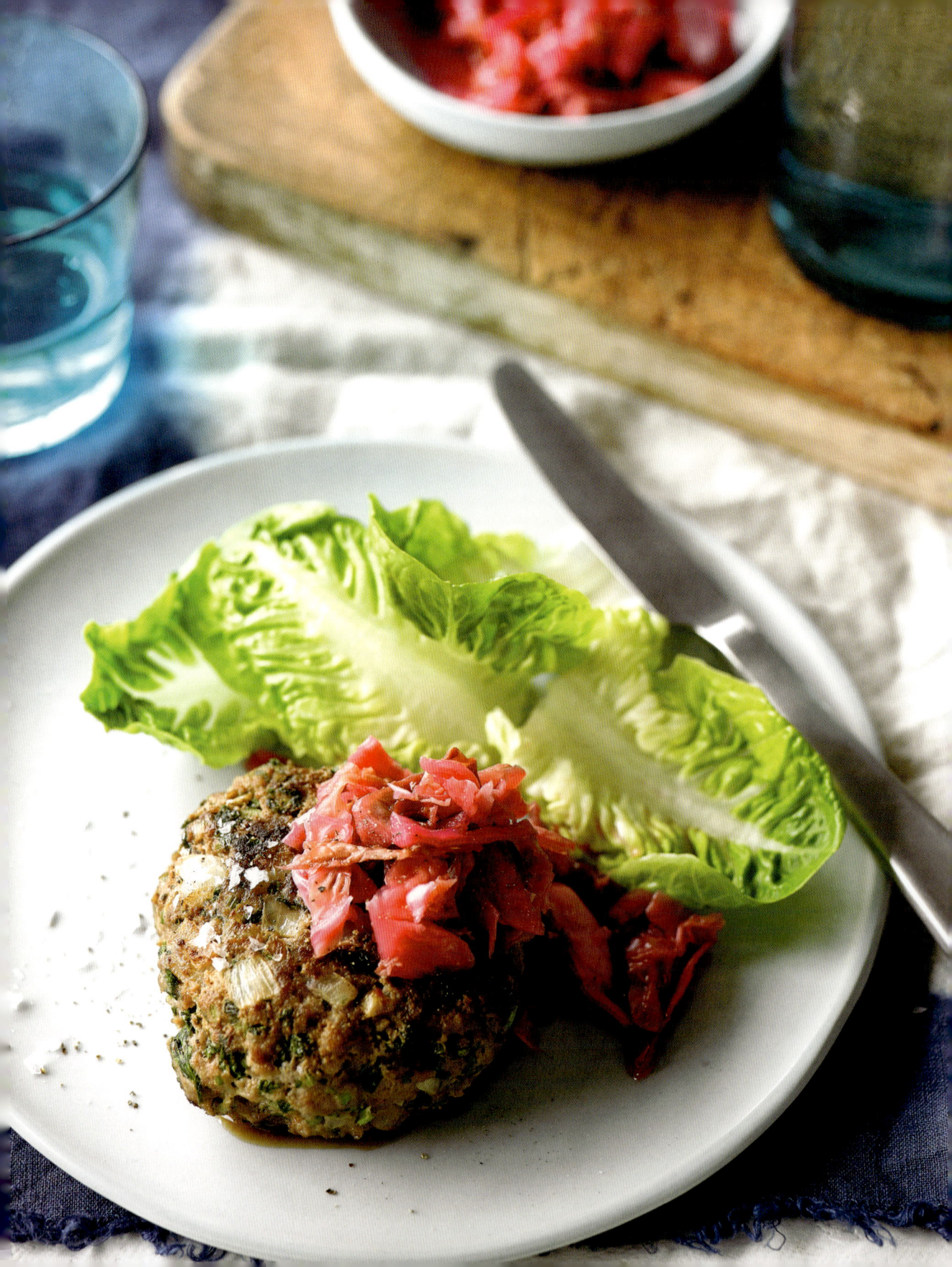

Burgers or Meatballs

Makes 4

This recipe is a go-to for any occasion – perfect for barbecues or kids' parties. The burgers are packed full of flavour and incredibly moist. This recipe shows there's no need to use breadcrumbs – an egg is all you need to bind the minced meat.

400 g mince (try lamb or beef, or a combination of both)

1 egg yolk

1 brown onion, roughly chopped

1 garlic clove, minced

1 teaspoon Dijon or seeded mustard

1 bunch fresh coriander leaves, roughly chopped

sea salt and ground black pepper

1 tablespoon coconut oil, for frying

green salad, to serve (optional)

sauerkraut, to serve (optional, see recipe on page 118)

1. In a large mixing bowl, combine the mince, egg yolk, onion, garlic, mustard, coriander, salt and pepper. Divide the mince into small meatballs or flatten to make 4 patties.

2. Heat the coconut oil in a large frying pan. Throw your patty onto the heat and cook for about 2–3 minutes on each side. (Times vary according to the thickness of the patty.) Once browned and just cooked, take the patty from the pan and let it rest. Serve with a green salad or sauerkraut if you like. Enjoy.

Crispy Skin Barramundi with Pico de Gallo

Serves 4

Pico de gallo is a fresh Mexican salsa that goes perfectly with fish. This dish can be prepared in no time at all and looks awesome on the table. Colour, nutrition and summer vibes – you can't go wrong!

4 × 200 g barramundi fillets, skin on

2 tablespoons coconut oil

Pico de Gallo

2 tomatoes, finely diced

½ bunch fresh coriander leaves, chopped

½ red onion, finely chopped

1 long red chilli, finely chopped

1 tablespoon lemon juice, plus extra to serve

3 tablespoons avocado or olive oil

sea salt and ground black pepper

1. Kick off this recipe by preparing the pico de gallo. Mix the tomato, coriander, onion, chilli, lemon juice and avocado oil together in a bowl. Season to taste, then set aside and focus on the fish.

2. To prepare the barramundi, season the fillets with salt and pepper. Put the coconut oil in a large frying pan over a medium-high heat. When it's hot, pop the fillets in skin side down and cook for 3 minutes, or until golden brown, then flip them with a spatula and cook for a further 3 minutes, until the flesh is completely opaque right through.

3. Serve alongside the pico de gallo.

TIP: This dish is delicious with our garlic aioli. Check out the recipe on page 129.

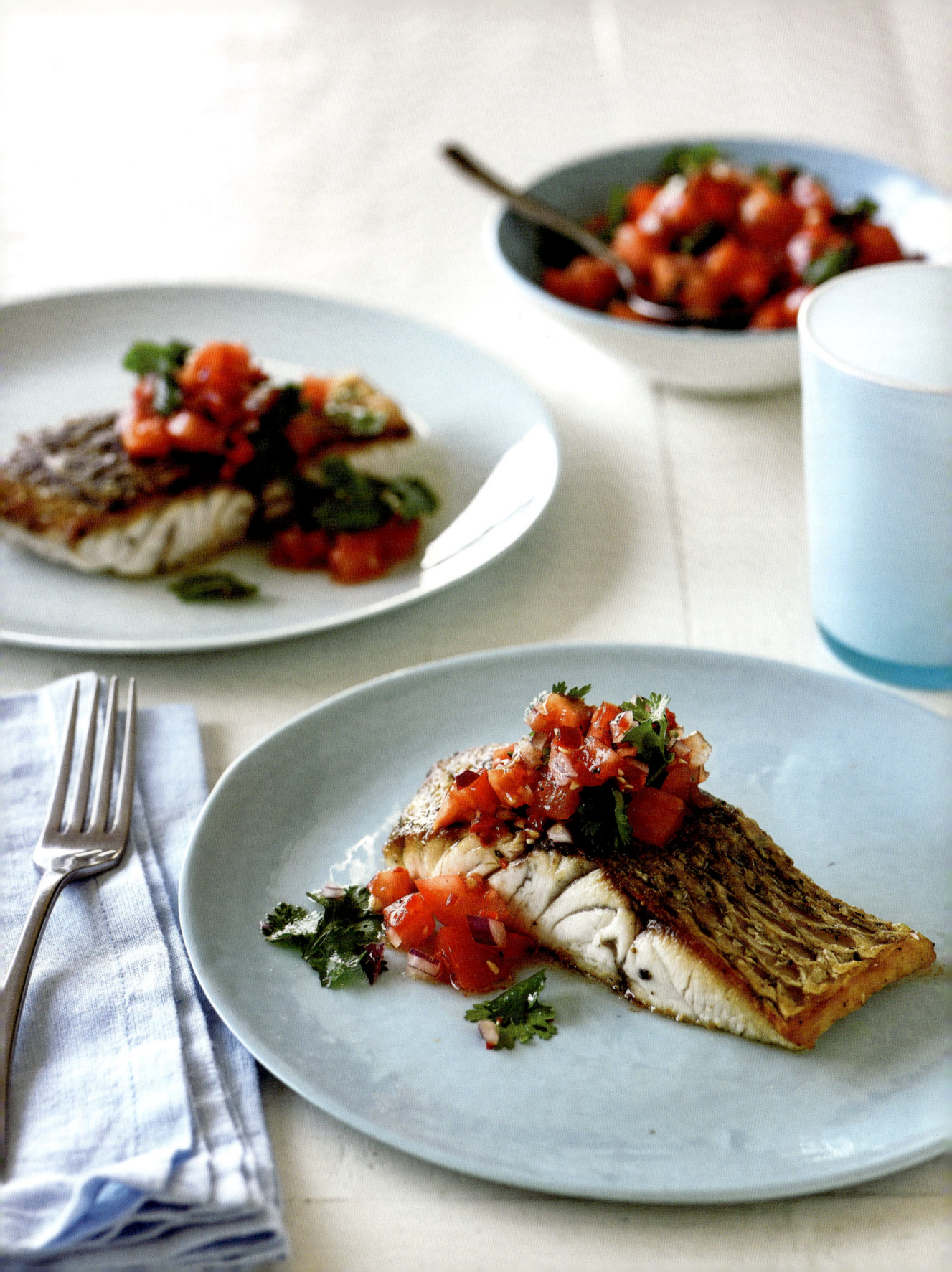

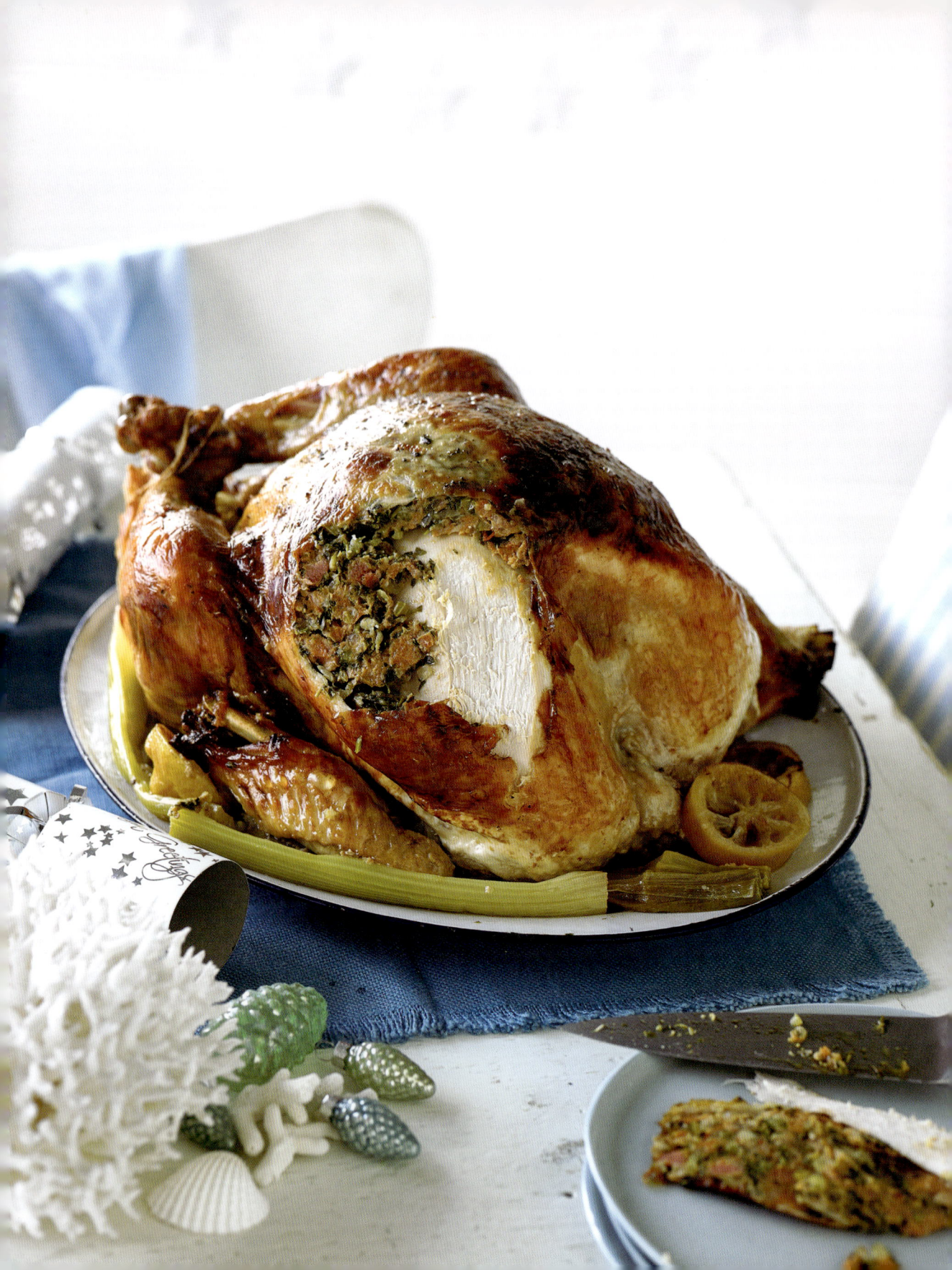

Christmas Turkey with Chorizo Stuffing

Serves 8

Christmas Day needs a roast bird. With this recipe you can have it with stuffing, just like you love and remember, but with none of the guilt. Yum.

4 leeks, green ends trimmed, halved lengthwise

4 stalks celery

4 lemons, thickly sliced into rounds

4 kg turkey

100 g butter, softened

2 cups white wine

2 cups chicken stock

sea salt and ground black pepper

Chorizo Stuffing

50 g butter

1 large red onion, finely chopped

1 stalk celery, finely chopped

6 fresh chorizo sausages, meat removed from casings

¼ cup finely chopped tarragon

¼ cup lemon thyme leaves

¼ cup chopped flat-leaf parsley

1. To make the chorizo stuffing, melt the butter in a large frying pan over a medium heat, then add the onion and celery. Cook, stirring occasionally, for 3 minutes, then transfer to a large, heat-proof bowl. Let them cool, then add all the remaining ingredients and mix well. Season to taste, then set aside.

2. Preheat your oven to 180°C. Arrange the leek and celery in a large, deep roasting pan, then top them with half the lemon slices.

3. Rinse the turkey inside and out, then pat it dry. Rest the turkey on top of the veggies, then season inside the cavity and fill with the remaining lemon slices.

4. Carefully push your fingertips underneath the skin that covers the turkey's breast meat to form a large pocket. Fill the pocket with the chorizo stuffing, covering the breast flesh evenly. Season the top of the turkey, then spread the butter all over the skin. Tie the legs together.

5. Pour the wine and stock into the pan. Cover the turkey with a double sheet of baking paper, then a double sheet of foil. Bake for 3 hours, or until the juices run clear when a skewer is inserted into the thickest part of the leg. Remove the foil and baking paper and cook for 30 minutes to brown.

6. Let the turkey rest in the pan, covered with 2 thick tea towels, for at least 20 minutes, then carve and serve with vegetables.

Garlic and Rosemary Focaccia

Serves 6

Paleo bread can be as tasty as the whole-wheat versions – this delicious and fragrant side dish pairs nicely with any of our roasted mains.

6 eggs, at room temperature

½ cup coconut milk

1 tablespoon lemon juice

⅔ cup coconut flour

1 teaspoon baking powder

sea salt and ground black pepper

3 garlic cloves, thinly sliced

2 tablespoons fresh rosemary leaves

25 g butter, melted

1. Preheat your oven to 200°C, then grease a 26 cm × 16 cm cake tin and line it with baking paper.
2. Whisk the eggs, coconut milk and lemon juice together in a large bowl. Add the coconut flour and baking powder and stir until well combined. The mixture will be soft and sticky. Season with salt, then spoon the batter into the cake tin and level the surface.
3. Press the garlic slices and rosemary all over the top of the focaccia, then drizzle it with the melted butter and season with salt and pepper.
4. Put the focaccia in the oven and bake for 25 minutes, or until golden. When it's cooked, a skewer inserted in the centre should come out clean. Let it stand in the tin for 5 minutes, then transfer to a chopping board. Slice and serve warm.

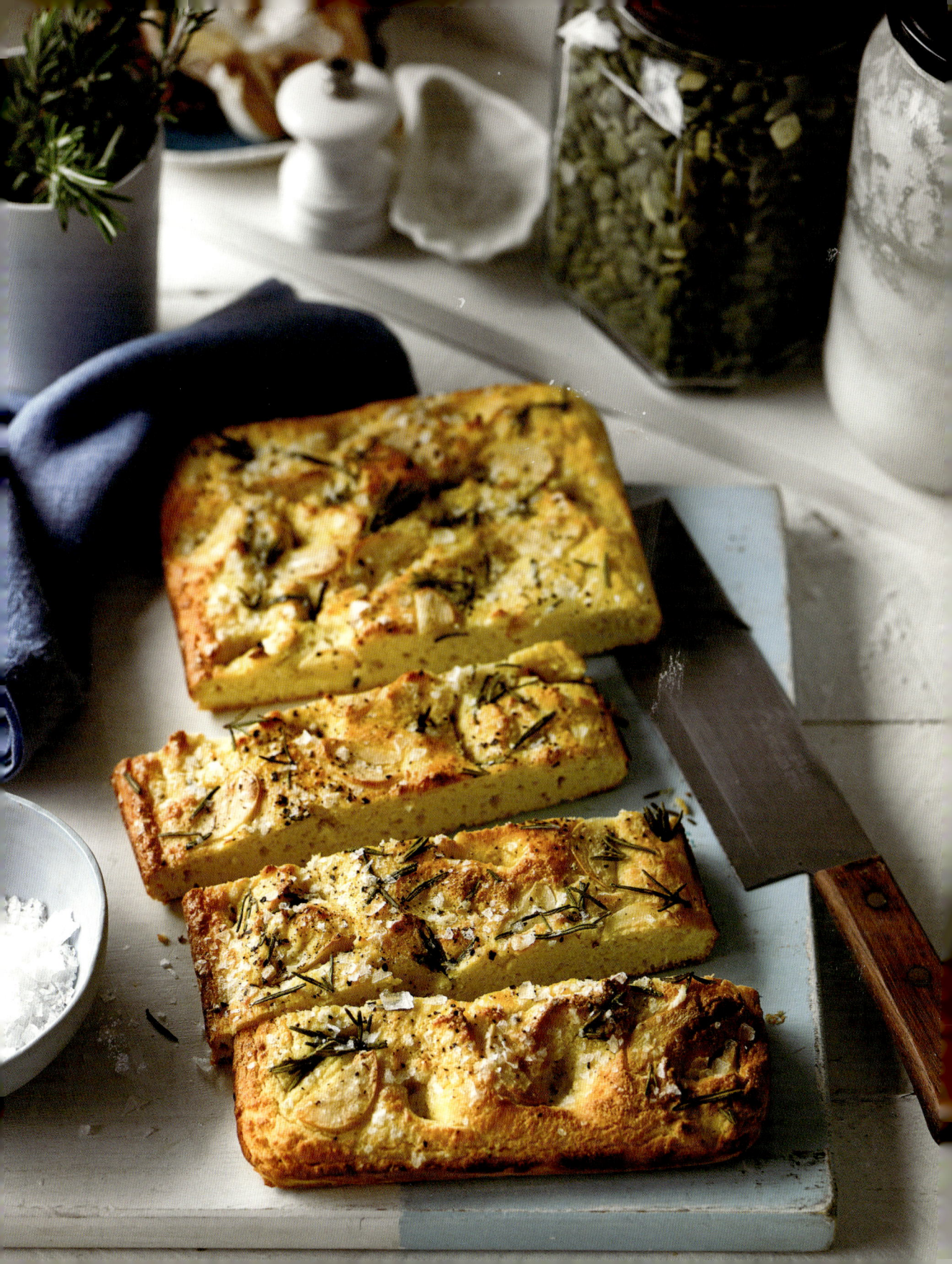

Mini Meatloaves with Avo Smash

Makes 12

These little meatloaves make a great dish when you have visitors – they look amazing on the plate and are an easy breakfast option, too!

12 round slices pancetta

1 tablespoon chia seeds

500 g beef mince

½ cup chopped flat-leaf parsley

2 tablespoons chopped oregano

2 tablespoons thyme leaves

1 garlic clove, crushed

2 Roma tomatoes, sliced

Avo Smash

2 zucchini, thickly sliced

400 g cauliflower florets

200 g broccoli florets

1 avocado

2 tablespoons avocado oil

finely grated zest and juice of
  1 small lemon

sea salt and ground black pepper

1. Preheat your oven to 200°C, then grease a 12-hole muffin pan and line each pan hole with a piece of pancetta.
2. Whisk the chia seeds with 2 tablespoons of water and set aside for 20 minutes, or until the seeds are plump and translucent.
3. Combine the chia mixture in a bowl with the mince, herbs and garlic, then season to taste. Divide the mixture evenly among the holes in the muffin pan. Top each mini loaf with a slice of tomato.
4. Bake for 30 minutes, or until the meatloaves are golden brown and cooked through when tested in the centre with a skewer.
5. Meanwhile, to make the avo smash, steam the zucchini, cauliflower and broccoli for 6–8 minutes, or until just tender. Transfer to a large, heat-proof bowl and add the remaining ingredients. Mash them roughly together and then season to taste.
6. Serve the hot mini meatloaves with the avo smash.

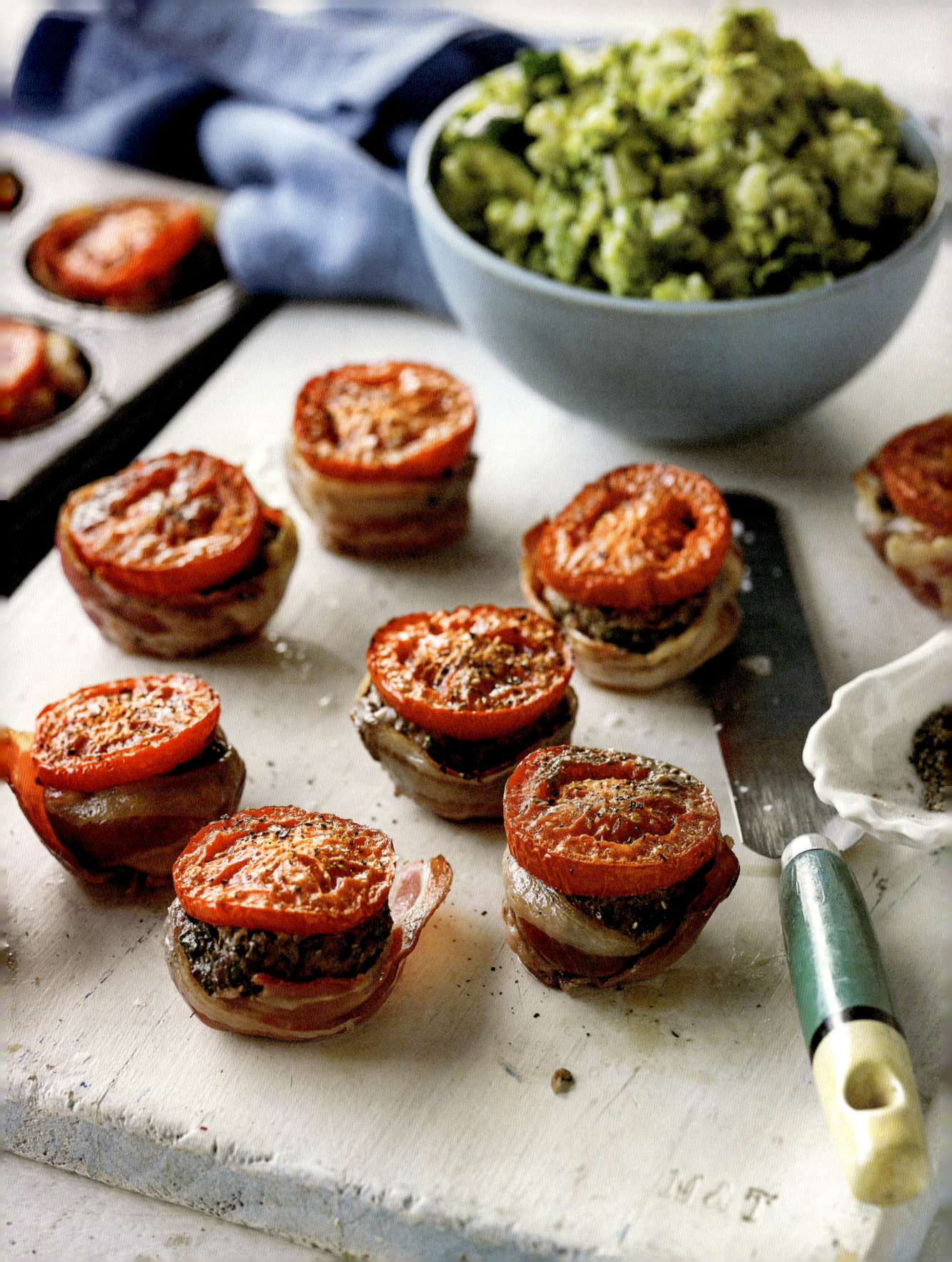

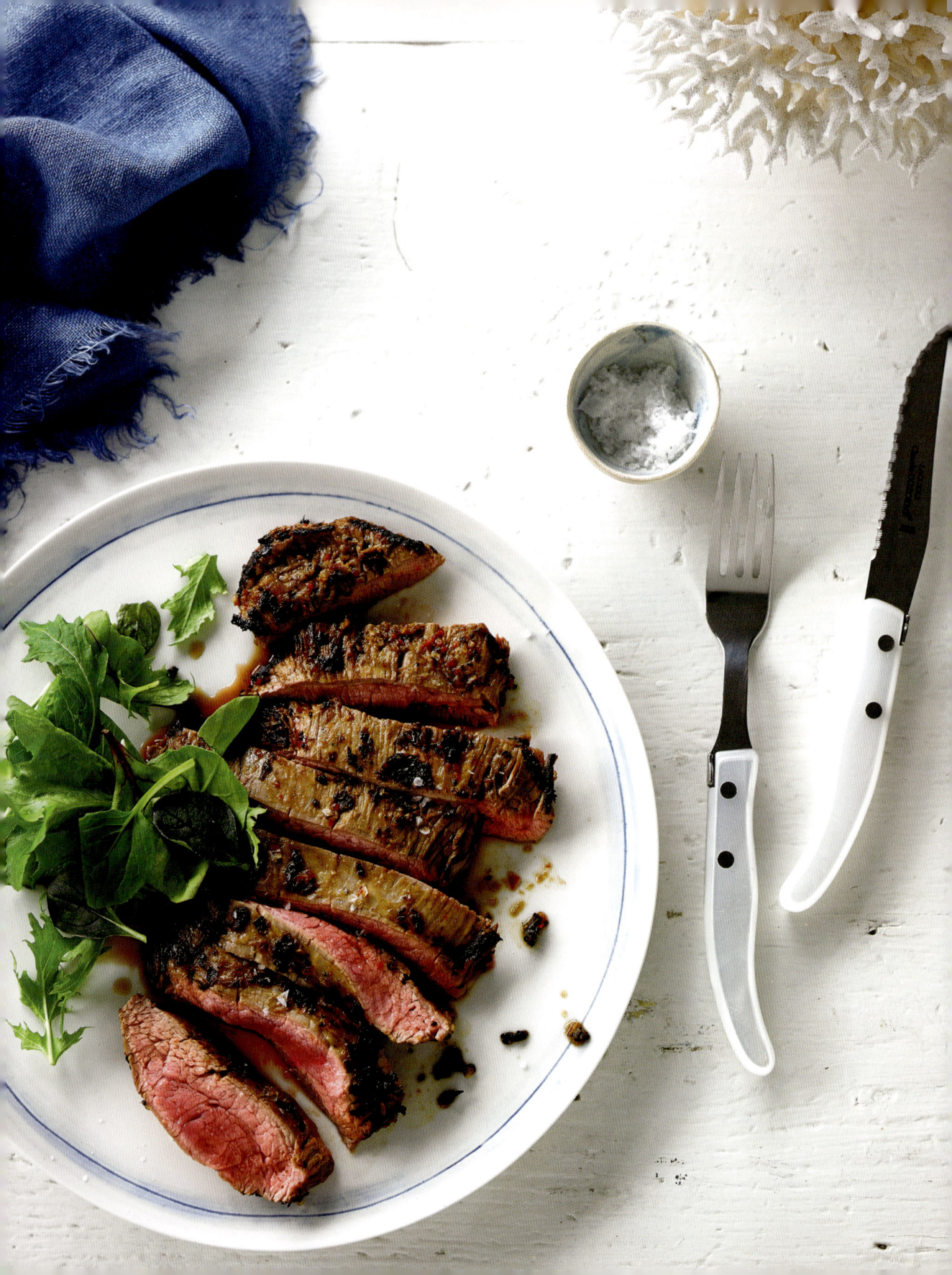

Kiwi Marinated Skirt Steak

Serves 4

Kiwis are clever little things . . . they possess an enzyme that helps to tenderise tough cuts of meat. Skirt is an exceptional cut of meat and affordable too, but it can be tough if you don't treat it right. Let it marinate for around two hours, but don't leave it too long, or it will become mushy.

2 long red chillis, seeded and roughly chopped

3 garlic cloves, finely chopped

2 teaspoons cumin seeds

¼ cup coconut oil

4 skirt steaks

4 kiwi fruit, peeled and smashed

sea salt and ground black pepper

mixed leaf salad, to serve

1. Using a mortar and pestle, pound the chilli, garlic and cumin seeds with a pinch of salt until they form a paste.

2. Put the coconut oil in a frying pan over a medium heat. When it's hot, add the paste and stir for 30–60 seconds, or until fragrant, before taking it off the heat, then set it aside to cool.

3. Put the steaks in a zip-lock bag or airtight container. Pour the marinade over the steaks, add the kiwi flesh and mix thoroughly, then pop it in the fridge for 2 hours.

4. Put a large frying pan over a high heat. When it's hot, pop the steaks in the pan and cook them for 3–4 minutes on each side, or until they're cooked the way you like them. Take them out of the pan, season and let them rest for 5 minutes, then serve and enjoy.

Crispy Fish Tacos with Guacamole

Serves 4

This is a wicked summer crowd-pleaser – with none of the carbs and sugar traditionally associated with tacos. Instead of the carb-heavy corn taco shell, we use lettuce cups to enjoy these babies!

500 g flathead fillets, skinned and pin-boned

sea salt

coconut oil, for deep-frying

8 butter or iceberg lettuce leaves

2 lemon cheeks

Crumb Coating

2 eggs

60 g tapioca flour

1 cup almond meal

Guacamole

1 avocado, roughly diced

1 small red chilli, seeded and roughly chopped

½ red onion, finely diced

1 garlic clove, finely chopped

2 tablespoons fresh coriander leaves, chopped

1 teaspoon ground cumin

1 teaspoon sweet paprika

1 tablespoon olive oil

juice of 1 lime

1. To make the guacamole, combine all of the ingredients in a small bowl. Set aside, ready to serve in your lettuce cup tacos with the fish.

2. To prepare your crumb coating, whisk the eggs in a bowl with 3 tablespoons of water, then set aside. Put the tapioca flour in another bowl, and the almond meal in a third bowl.

3. Cut the flathead fillets into eight even portions and season them with a little salt. Dust the fish pieces lightly with the tapioca flour, dip them in the egg mixture, and then press them firmly in the almond meal until both sides are coated.

4. Put the coconut oil in a wok or large saucepan and heat it to 160°C. To make sure the oil is at the right temperature, drop in a small piece of fish. It should bubble instantly around the edges.

5. Fry the fish in batches, for about 90 seconds per batch, or until cooked through. Drain the fish on paper towel and season with salt.

6. Put the fish in a lettuce cup, give it a good dollop of guacamole and squeeze a little lemon juice over the top, then wrap to form the tacos.

TIP: We use flathead caught in New South Wales or Victoria, which get the tick from the Sustainable Seafood Guide. Try to steer clear of their relatives from Tassie or Queensland.

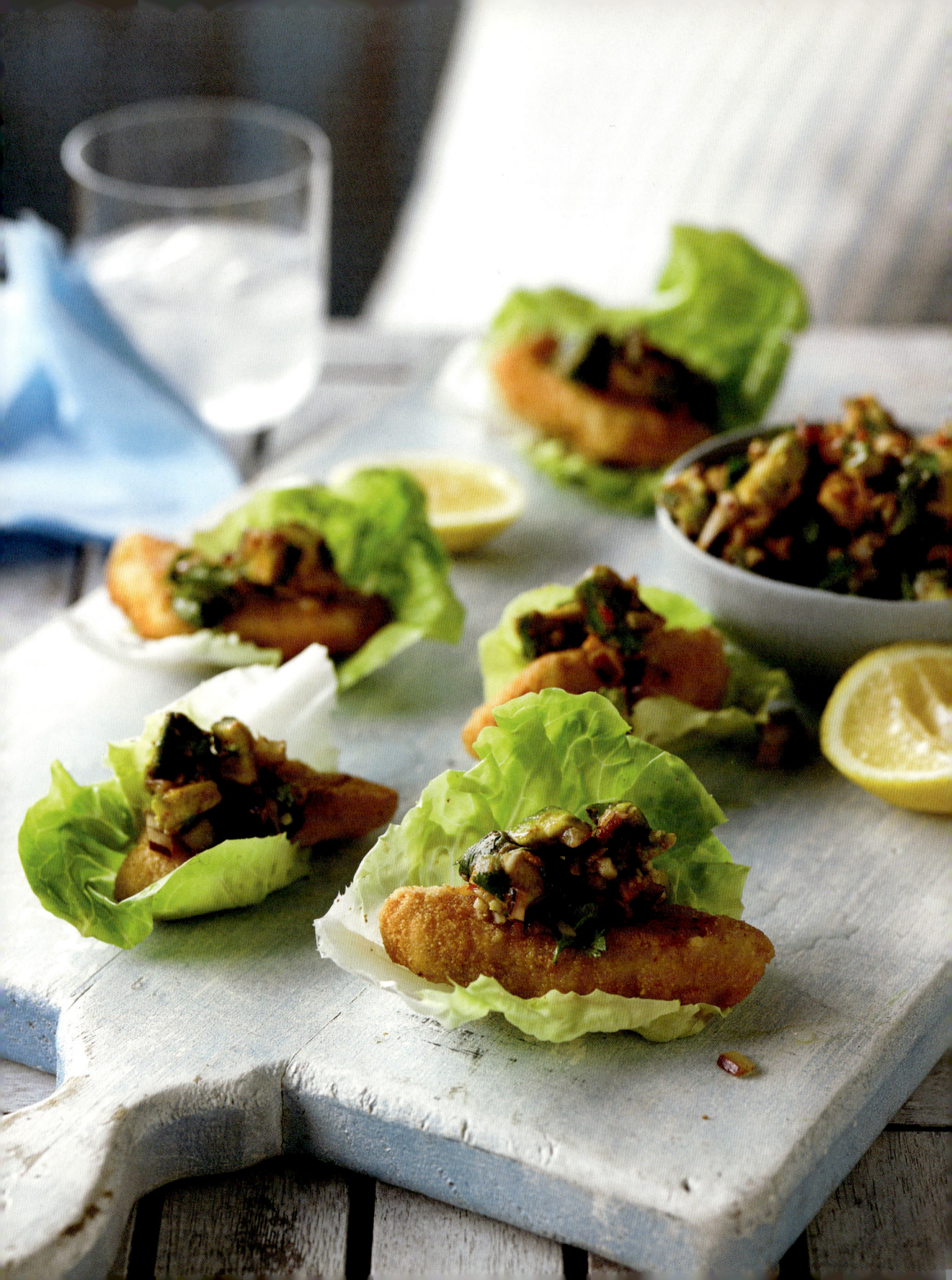

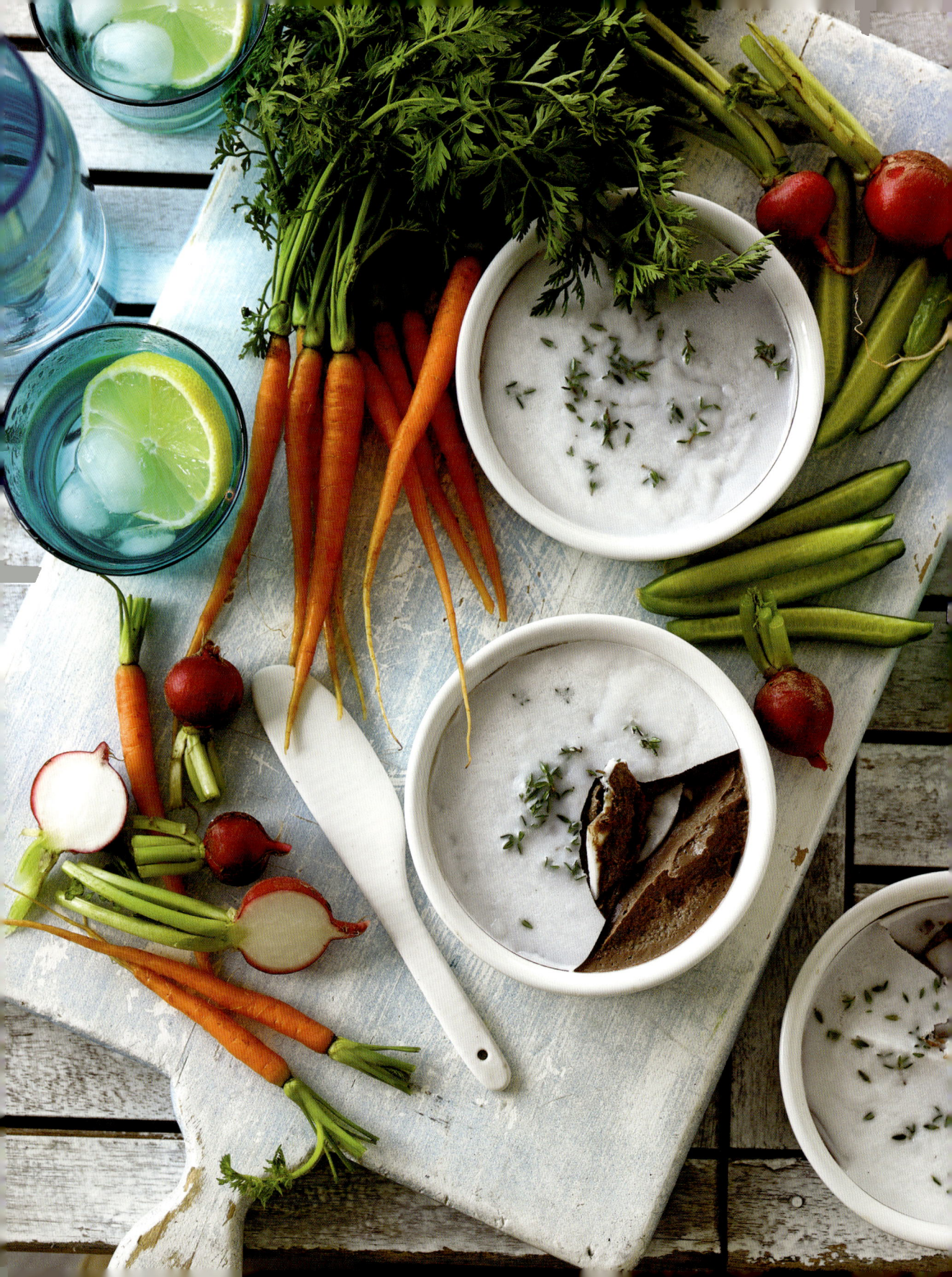

Luke and Scott's Pâté

Makes 300 ml

Pâté is a perfect snack or entree that delivers an intense hit of nutrients and vitamins. Organ meats, such as liver, are extremely nutrient-dense and should be consumed regularly for optimal health. Our early ancestors valued offal over lean meat, as it provided the biggest nutritional return from their hunt.

1 small brown onion, finely chopped

2–3 garlic cloves, finely minced

½ cup coconut oil (optional), plus extra for frying

400 g chicken livers, sinew and discoloured bits removed

1 sprig rosemary

2 sprigs thyme, plus extra leaves (optional)

¼ teaspoon ground nutmeg

1 teaspoon Dijon mustard

1 teaspoon lemon juice

½ cup red wine

sea salt and ground black pepper

1. In a frying pan, sauté the onion, garlic and a little coconut oil with the livers over a medium heat until the livers are browned and the onion has softened.

2. Add the rosemary, thyme, nutmeg, mustard, lemon juice and wine to the pan and cook until half the liquid has evaporated.

3. Transfer the cooked liver and onion mixture to a food processor, discarding the herb sprigs first, and blend, adding the pan juices gradually until it is smooth, then season to taste.

4. Put the mixture in a shallow dish or small individual ramekins. If you wish, you can top the pâté with melted coconut oil and sprinkle with extra thyme leaves. The coconut oil will form an airtight seal once chilled. Pop the pâté in the fridge for 2–3 hours.

5. Serve with chopped radish, baby carrots and baby cucumber or simply by the spoonful.

Tea-Smoked Trout Blini

Makes 20

These AMAZING blini make the perfect paleo hors d'oeuvre when you've got guests coming round and you want to serve something a little special.

½ cup dried tea-leaves

½ cup uncooked jasmine rice

1 tablespoon allspice berries

300 g skinless, boneless ocean trout

1 large beetroot, peeled, coarsely grated

1 tablespoon finely grated fresh horseradish

¼ cup dill leaves

2 tablespoons hemp seed oil

black lumpfish caviar, to serve

micro herbs, to serve

Blini

½ cup almond meal

¼ cup arrowroot

1 teaspoon baking powder

2 spring onions, thinly sliced

2 eggs, lightly whisked

1 tablespoon coconut milk

sea salt and ground black pepper

coconut oil, for cooking

1. To make the blini, combine all the ingredients except the coconut oil in a bowl, then season to taste. Melt a little coconut oil in a large frying pan over a medium heat. Pour 3 teaspoonful measures of the batter into the pan and repeat until you have 5 or 6 blini. Cook the blini for 1–2 minutes on each side, or until they are golden. Transfer to a wire rack, then repeat until you've used up all the mixture. Set the cooked blini aside to cool.

2. To smoke the trout, line a large wok with 4 sheets of foil. Combine the tea-leaves, rice and allspice in a bowl, then pour them into the wok and spread them out to form a layer 2 cm thick. Set a greased wire rack over the tea-leaf mixture, making sure there is a 4 cm gap between the tea mixture and the rack. Turn on your stove's extractor fan and open all doors and windows, then put the wok over a high heat. Let the tea mixture cook for 2–3 minutes, or until you see it start to smoke.

3. Put the fish on the wire rack in the wok and cover it with a tight-fitting lid. Let it smoke for 10–12 minutes, or until it's just cooked. Take the wok off the heat and let it stand, uncovered, for 5 minutes, then remove the fish and, using a fork, pull the flesh apart into thick flakes and set aside.

4. Put the beetroot, horseradish, dill and hemp seed oil in a bowl and mix to combine. Season to taste.

5. Put the blini on a large serving platter and spoon the beetroot mixture over them. Top with smoked trout, caviar and micro herbs.

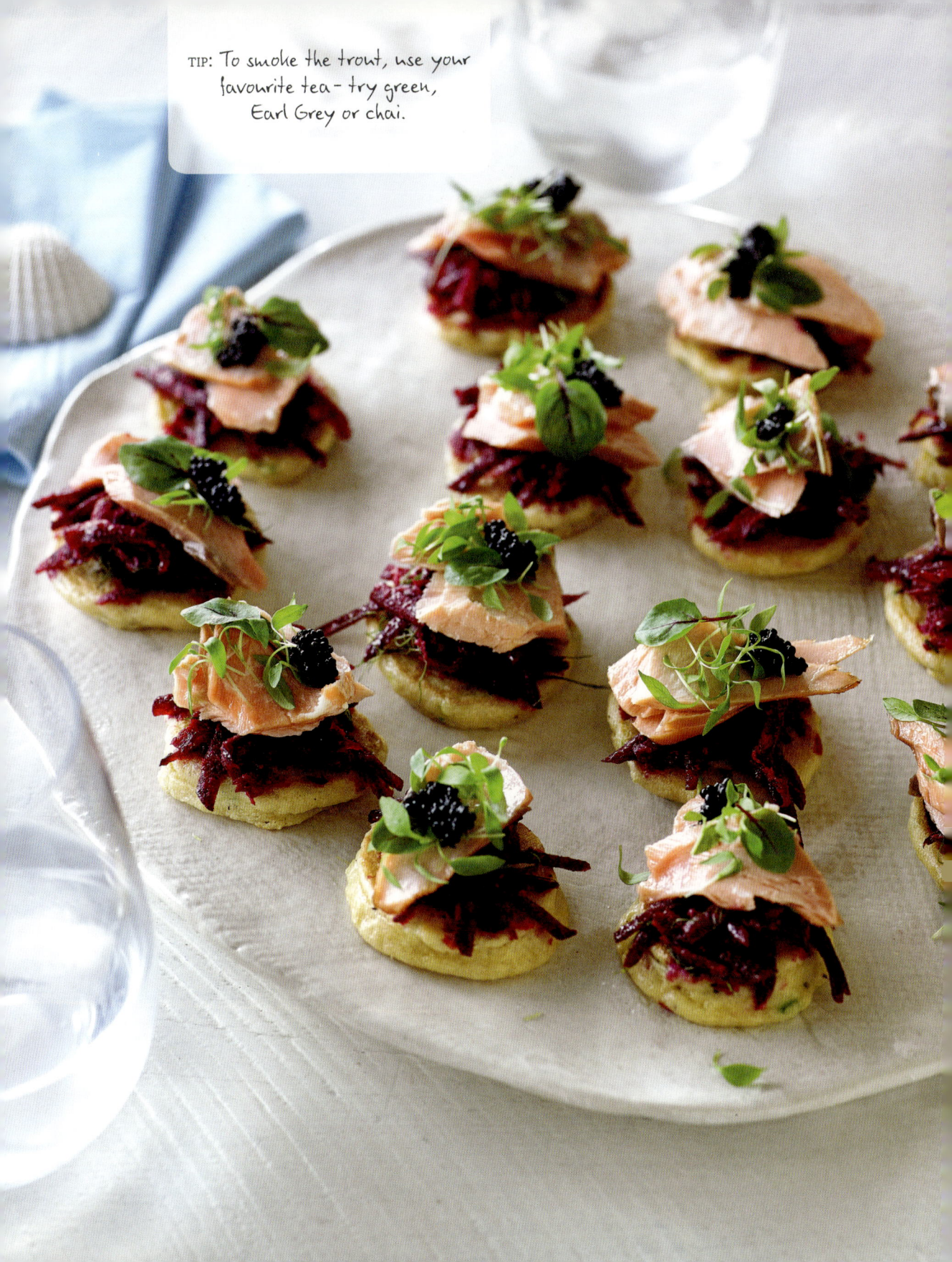

TIP: To smoke the trout, use your favourite tea – try green, Earl Grey or chai.

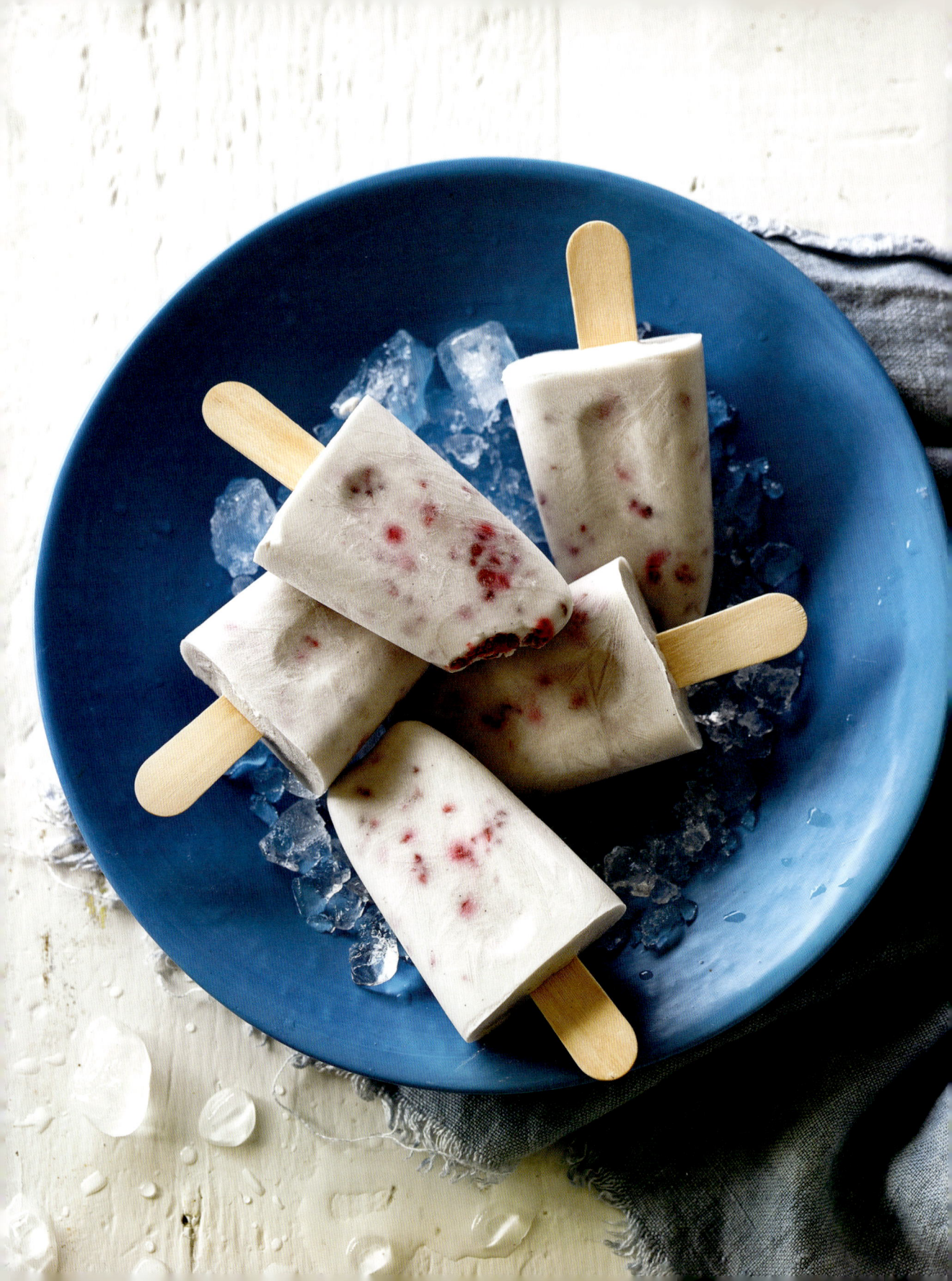

Icy Poles

Makes 6

The kids will absolutely love this quick and simple recipe. They're great for a treat on a hot summer's day.

400 ml can coconut cream

½ cup fresh or frozen raspberries, roughly mashed with a fork

1 vanilla bean, seeds scraped

1. In a bowl, gently combine the coconut cream, raspberries and vanilla seeds.

2. Carefully pour the mixture into icy-pole moulds, inserting sticks if required, and put them in the freezer for 2–3 hours, or until you're ready to eat them.

Mango Lime Chia Pudding

Serves 2

These little puddings have summer written all over them. They're fresh, zesty and addictive. Simple to make and so quick to devour, you may want to double up the quantities on this one.

1 ripe mango, diced

2.5 cm piece ginger, peeled, sliced

1 cup coconut milk

1 teaspoon maple syrup or honey

juice of 1 lime

¼ cup chia seeds

½ cup flaked coconut, toasted

½ cup pistachios, toasted

1 teaspoon ground cinnamon, to dust

1. Combine the mango, ginger, coconut milk, maple syrup and lime juice in a food processor and blend until really smooth.
2. Pour the mixture into a bowl, add the chia seeds and whisk together to combine.
3. Pour the mixture into two 250 ml glasses. Let the puddings chill in the fridge for at least 3 hours, or overnight, then serve sprinkled with toasted coconut and pistachios and dusted with cinnamon.

TIP: Serve in clear glasses for extra effect.

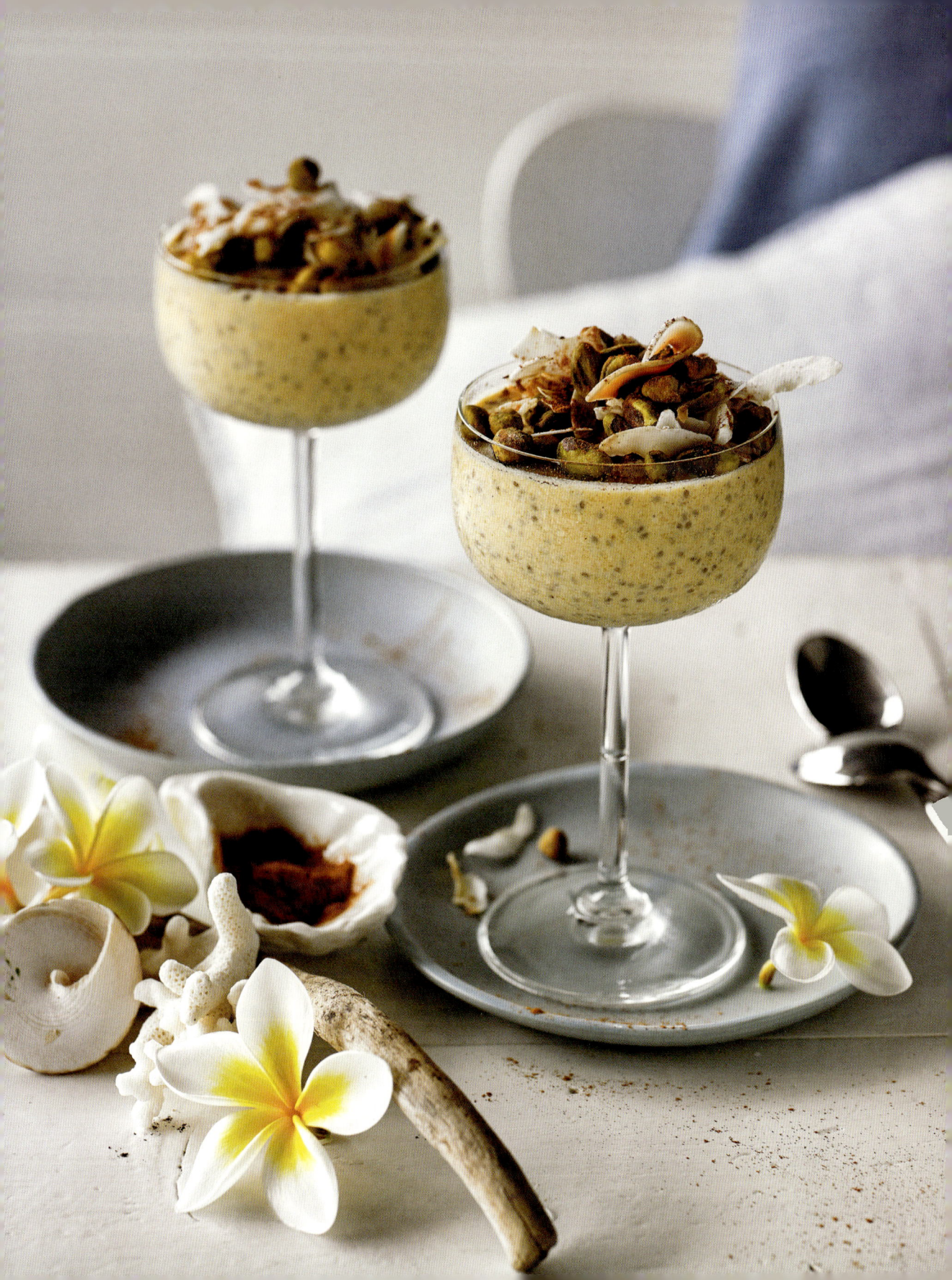

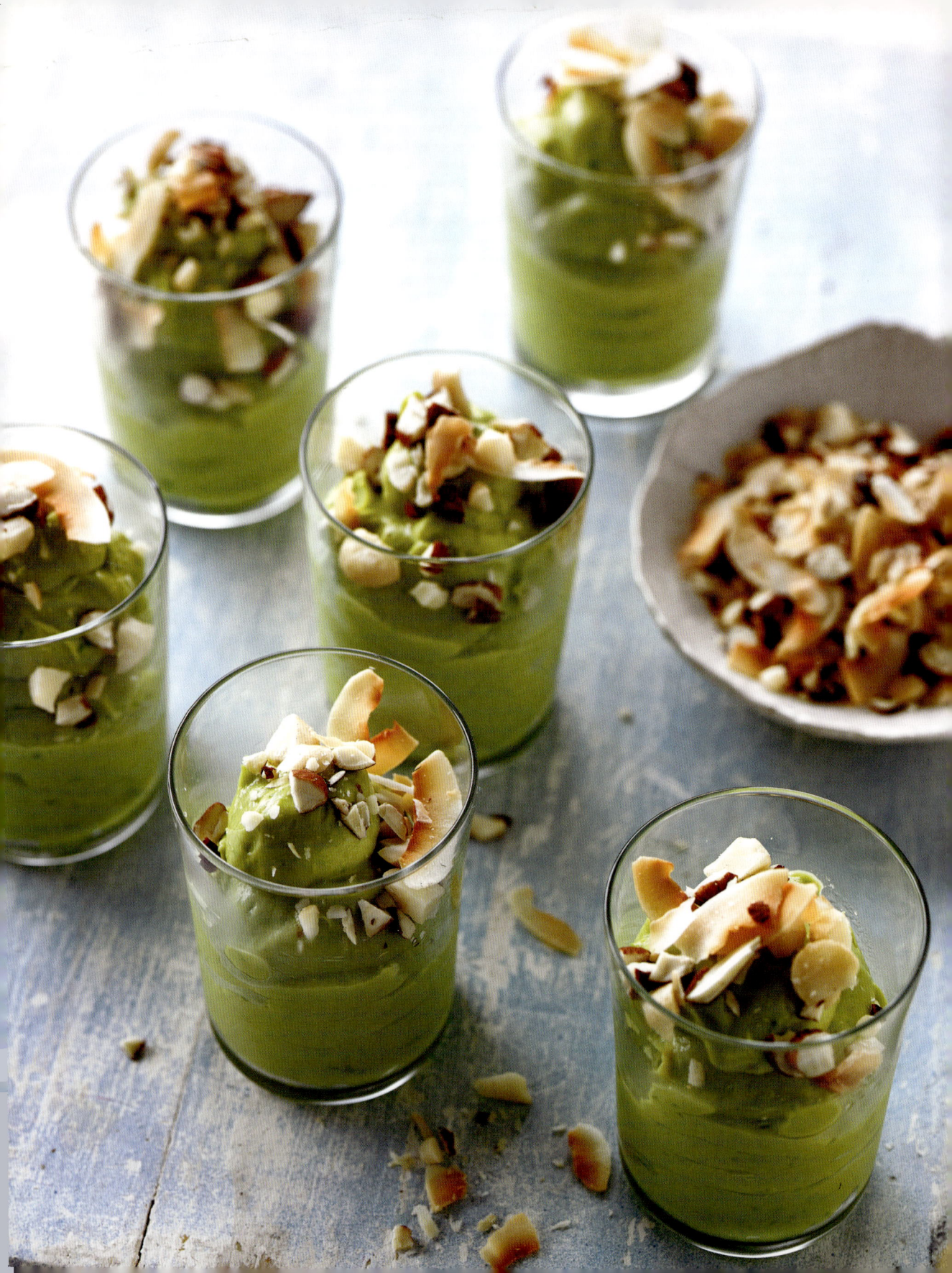

Lime Mousse with Toasted Nut Crumble

Serves 6

Avocado is a great source of good fat, and the lime juice and honey make this mousse tangy and sweet. It's a great summer dessert, as it's light and refreshing but still keeps you feeling full. Add some different nuts and seeds to the crumble if you'd like to mix it up.

5 ripe avocados, halved, stones removed and peeled

½ cup lime juice

zest of 4 limes

½ cup honey

2 tablespoons coconut oil

2 teaspoons vanilla extract

½ teaspoon sea salt

¼ cup macadamias, finely chopped

¼ cup almonds, finely chopped

¼ cup shredded coconut

1. Combine the avocados, lime juice and zest, honey, coconut oil, vanilla and sea salt in a food processor or blender and process until smooth. Add a little more honey if you'd like it sweeter.
2. Pour the mousse mixture into a bowl and put it in the fridge to chill.
3. Toast the macadamias, almonds and coconut, in a frying pan over a medium heat.
4. Serve the mousse with the nuts scattered over the top.

Salted Caramel Choc Fudge

Makes 8 pieces

Salted caramel is certainly very trendy these days, and for good reason. We can't get enough of that perfect combination of sweet and savoury together in one bite. This salted caramel choc fudge is completely no fuss, as there is no baking needed!

1 cup macadamia nuts

12 dates, pitted

⅓ cup coconut oil, melted

1 teaspoon raw cacao powder

1 teaspoon vanilla extract

2 teaspoons salt

½ cup almond flakes, toasted

Chocolate Topping

¼ cup coconut oil

2 tablespoons raw cacao powder

1 tablespoon maple syrup
  or honey

2 tablespoons coconut milk

1 teaspoon vanilla extract

1. Soak the macadamias and dates in hot water for 10 minutes. While they are soaking, line a 16 cm square or rectangular cake tin with baking paper.

2. Put the macadamias, dates, coconut oil, cacao, vanilla and salt in a food processor, then process for 3–4 minutes, scraping the side as you go.

3. Add half of the toasted almond flakes to the food processor. Whiz a few more times until the almonds have been ground up and incorporated into the fudge mix. They don't have to be ground up super-fine, as it's good to have some texture coming through.

4. Scoop the fudge mixture out into the tin, then flatten and smooth the top with a spatula. Put the tin in the fridge while you make the chocolate topping.

5. To make the chocolate topping, melt the coconut oil with the cacao, maple syrup, coconut milk and vanilla.

6. Take the tin out of the fridge and pour the chocolate topping over the fudge. Spread it evenly with a spatula, then scatter the remaining toasted almonds over the top and put the tin back in the fridge for 2–3 hours. Cut into pieces before serving.

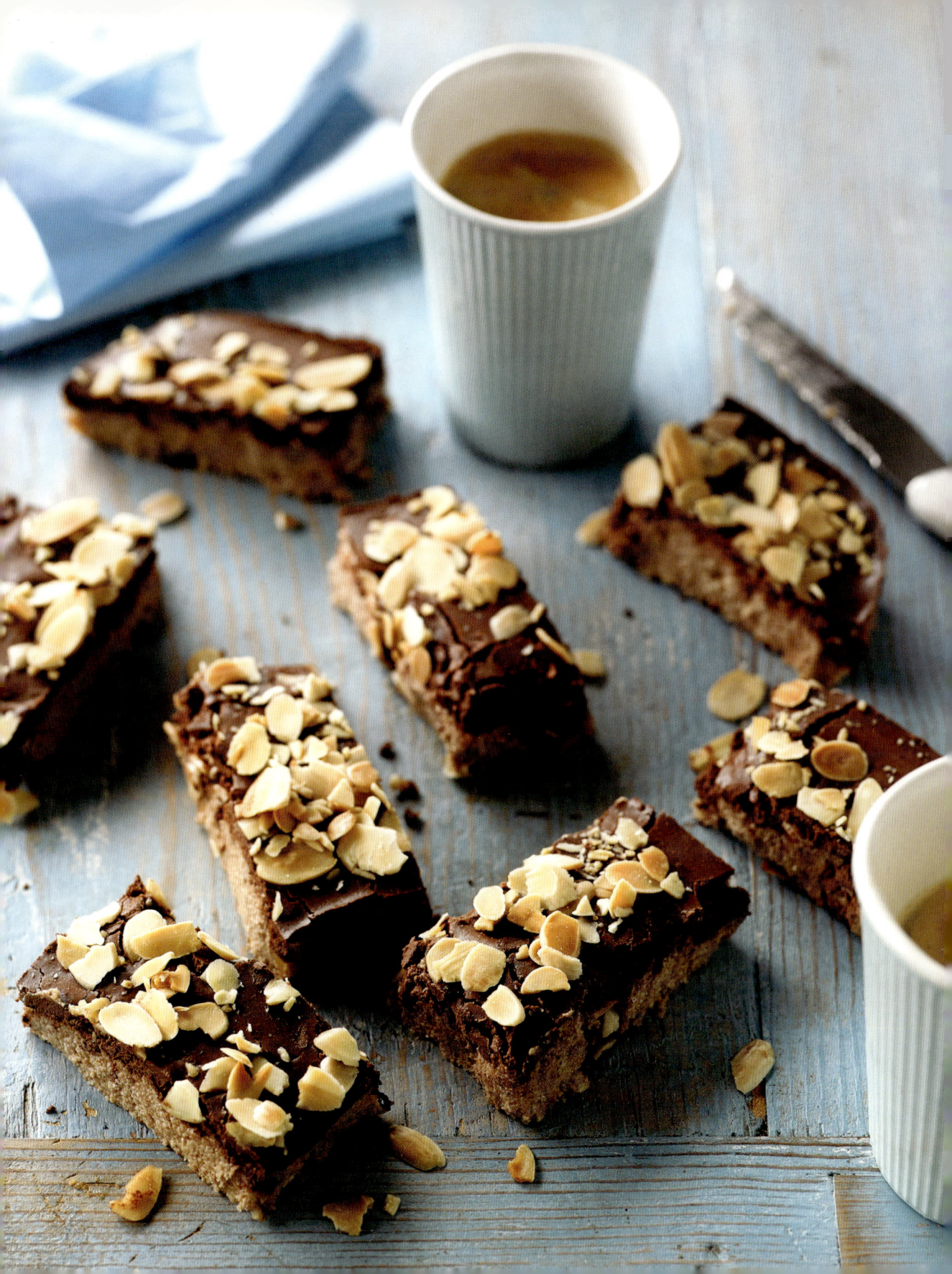

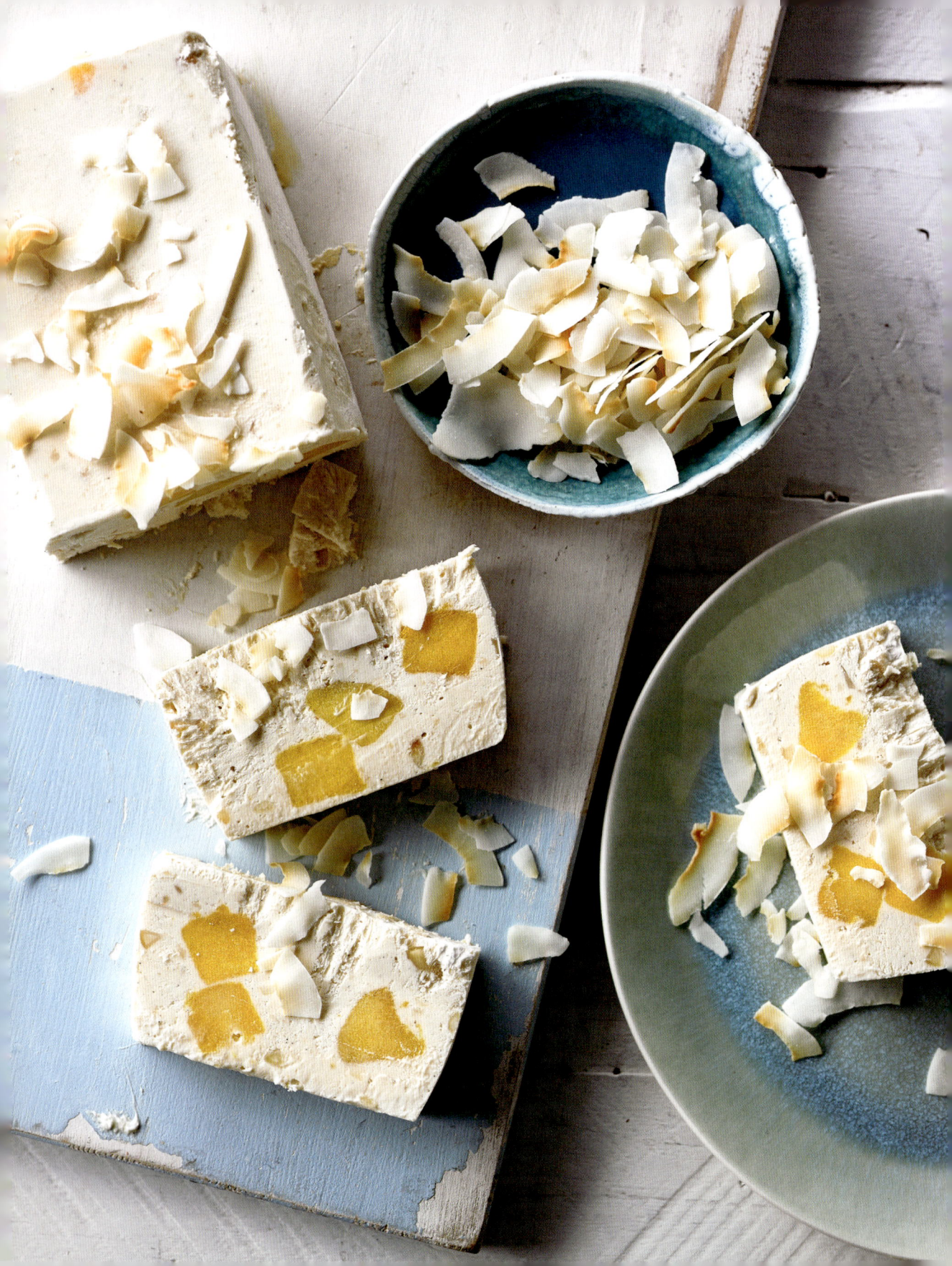

Coconut and Mango Semifreddo

Serves 10

Aussie summers really deliver the heat, and we know you want to reach for the ice-cream when the mercury is high. Instead, make this great clean dessert to cool yourself down. You'll need to plan ahead just a little – the cans of coconut cream go in the fridge overnight.

2 × 400 ml cans coconut cream

1 egg, at room temperature

2 egg yolks, at room temperature

⅓ cup maple syrup

2 vanilla beans, seeds scraped

½ cup macadamias, finely chopped and toasted

1 small mango, peeled, cheeks removed and chopped

½ cup flaked coconut, toasted

1. Chill the cans of coconut cream in the fridge overnight, so they'll be ready to go when you are.
2. Chill a mixing bowl in the freezer for half an hour, then line a 10 × 20 cm loaf tin with cling film.
3. Put the egg, egg yolks and maple syrup in another bowl, then whisk them using an electric mixer for 4 minutes, or until the mixture is pale and fluffy and has quadrupled in size.
4. Take the chilled bowl from the freezer. Open the chilled cans of coconut cream, then spoon the thick layer of cream off the top and into the chilled bowl. You will need 1½ cups of this firm cream. (You can use the leftover coconut milk in your breakfast smoothies.)
5. Using an electric mixer, whisk the chilled cream until soft peaks form. Fold through the vanilla seeds, macadamias and mango.
6. Fold one-third of the coconut cream mixture into the egg mixture until very well combined, then very gently fold in the remaining cream mixture until just combined. Do not over-mix. Spoon the mixture into the prepared tin and level the top. Freeze for 6 hours, or overnight if time permits.
7. Turn the semifreddo out onto a serving platter and top with the coconut flakes. Stand for 10 minutes before slicing and serving.

Red Velvet Celebration Cake

Serves 10

Birthdays and other celebrations are the easiest way to fall off the clean-eating wagon. Avoid that mistake by making this easy and impressive paleo cake instead!

150 g butter, at room temperature

¾ cup rice syrup

2 eggs, at room temperature

1 cup coconut flour

1½ cups arrowroot

2 tablespoons raw cacao powder

1 cup unsweetened almond milk

1 teaspoon bicarb soda

2 teaspoons baking powder

1 tablespoon apple cider vinegar

2 tablespoons red food colouring

250 g fresh raspberries

extra fresh raspberries, to serve

Lemon Buttercream

250 g unsalted butter, at room temperature

1 cup rice syrup

2 vanilla beans, seeds scraped

1 tablespoon finely grated lemon zest

1. Preheat your oven to 180°C, then grease two 20 cm round cake tins and line them with baking paper.

2. Using an electric mixer, whisk the butter and rice syrup together in a large bowl until pale and creamy. Whisk in the eggs one at a time, beating well after each addition, until well combined. Add the coconut flour, arrowroot, cacao and almond milk, and then slowly whisk until almost combined. Add the bicarb soda, baking powder, vinegar and food colouring and whisk until well combined.

3. Spoon the cake batter evenly between the tins and level the surfaces. Bake for 30 minutes, or until a skewer inserted in the centre comes out clean. Let stand in the tins for 5 minutes, then transfer the cakes to a wire rack to cool.

4. To make the lemon buttercream, use a handheld mixer to whisk the butter and rice syrup together for 2 minutes, or until pale and creamy. Add the vanilla seeds and lemon zest, then stir together until well combined.

5. Put one of the cakes on a serving platter. Spread the top with one-third of the lemon buttercream and top with the raspberries. Put the second cake on top and spread the top and sides with the remaining lemon buttercream.

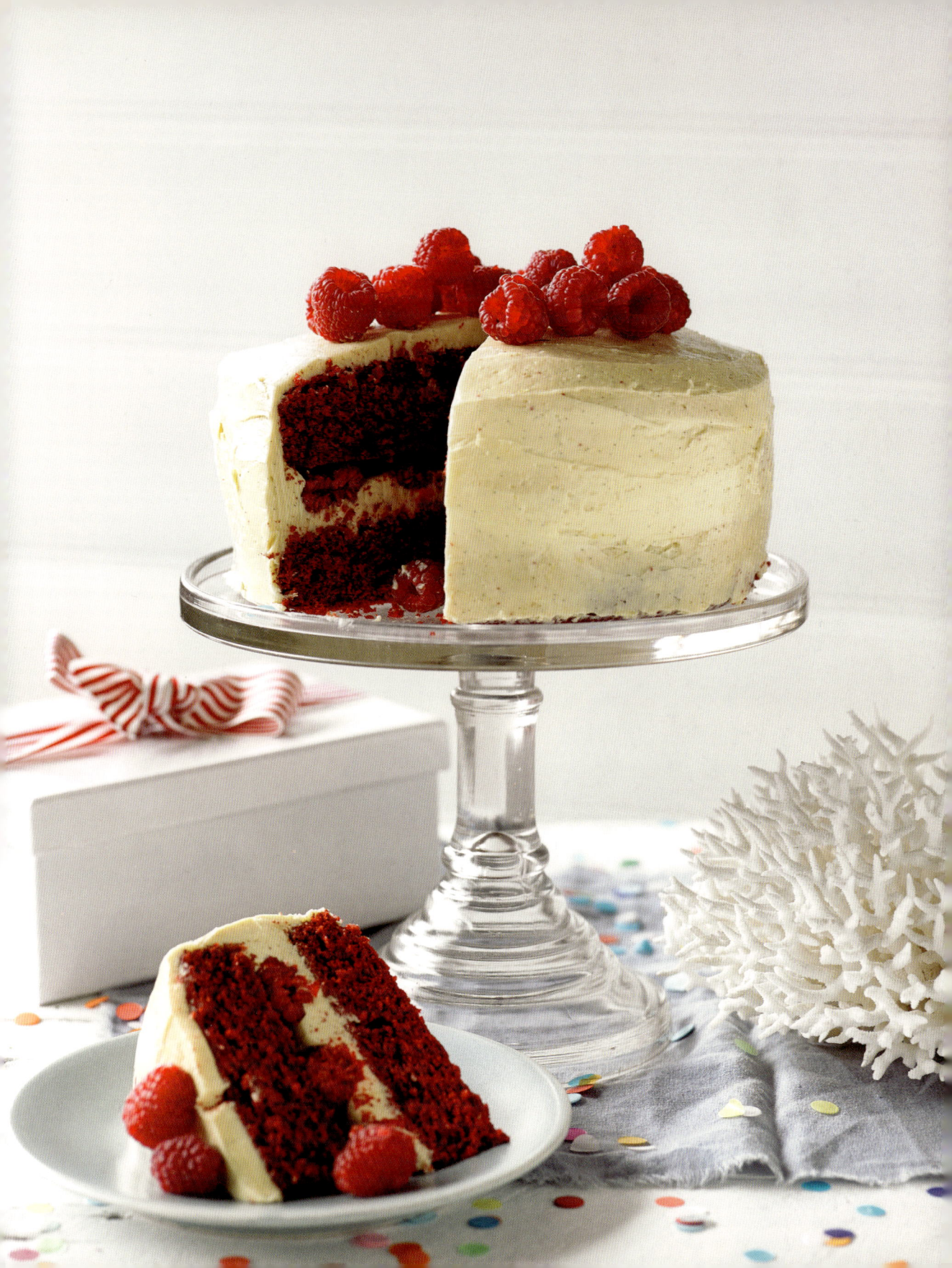

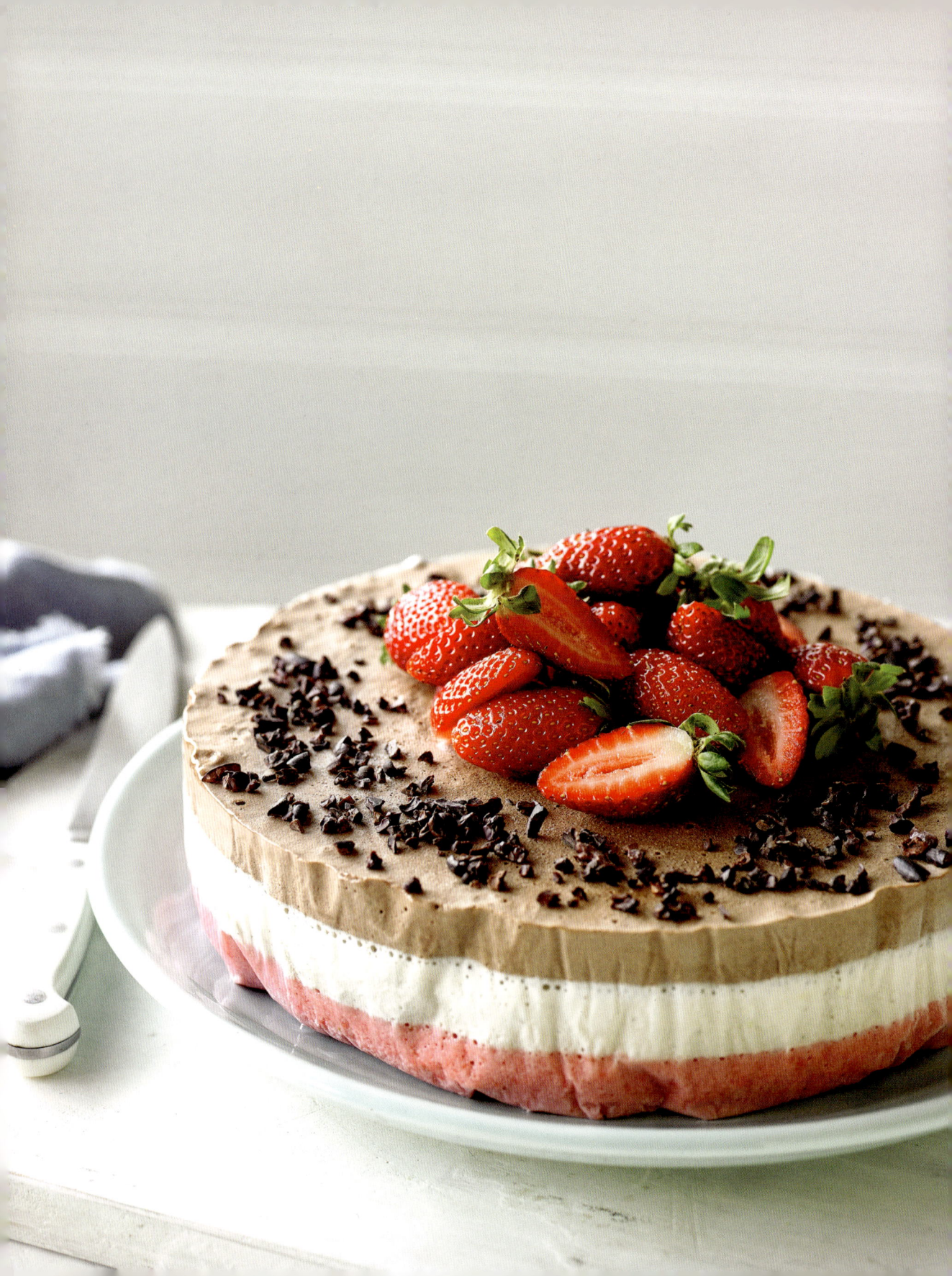

Neapolitan Ice-Cream Cake

Serves 12

Neapolitan has always been the classic flavour combo: strawberry, chocolate and vanilla. Here's our clean ice-cream cake version – all of the flavour, none of the nasties.

Strawberry Ice-Cream

250 g frozen strawberries,
  plus some fresh ones to serve

400 ml can coconut cream

¼ cup maple syrup

Vanilla Ice-Cream

2 frozen bananas, chopped

2 vanilla beans, seeds scraped

400 ml can coconut cream

¼ cup maple syrup

Chocolate Ice-Cream

2 frozen bananas, chopped

¼ cup raw cacao powder

400 ml can coconut cream

¼ cup maple syrup

raw cacao chips, to serve

1. Grease a 22 cm round springform cake tin and line it with baking paper.

2. To make the strawberry ice-cream, put the strawberries, coconut cream and maple syrup in a blender and blend until smooth, then pour into the cake tin. Freeze for 1 hour, or until very firm.

3. To make the vanilla ice-cream, put the bananas, vanilla seeds, coconut cream and maple syrup in a blender and blend until smooth. Pour over the firmly set strawberry ice-cream layer in the cake tin. Freeze for 1 hour, or until very firm.

4. To make the chocolate ice-cream, put the bananas, cacao, coconut cream and maple syrup in a blender and blend until smooth. Pour over the firmly set vanilla ice-cream layer in the cake tin. Freeze for 6 hours, or overnight if time permits.

5. Release the side of the cake tin and transfer the ice-cream cake to a serving plate. Top with the extra strawberries and the cacao chips. Let stand for 10 minutes before slicing and serving.

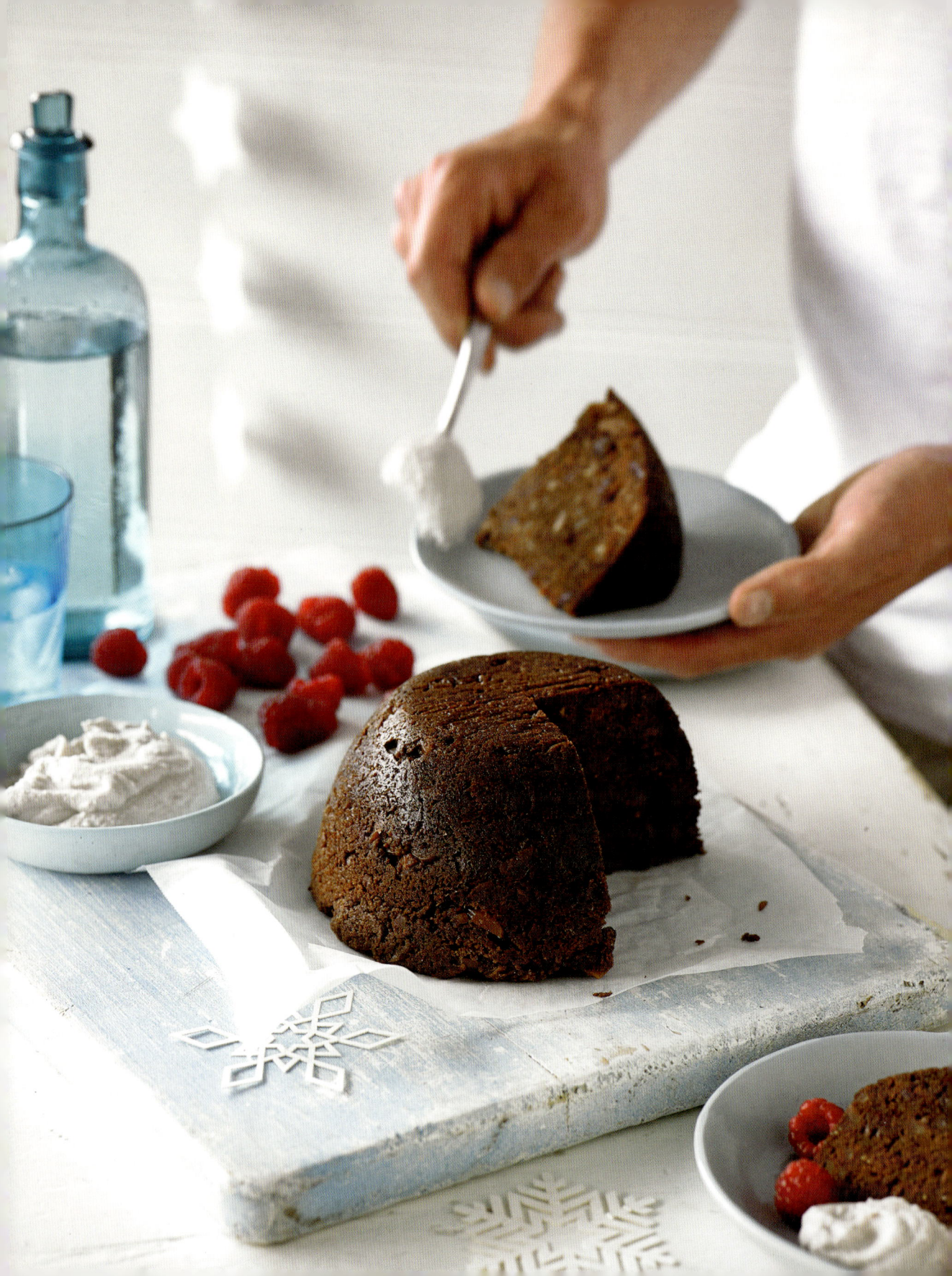

Christmas Pudding with Spiced Cream

Serves 8

It's not Christmas time without a delicious pudding – but there's no need for all that refined sugar and flour. Our pud is all goodness. You'll need to plan ahead just a little to make the spiced cream – the cans of coconut cream go in the fridge overnight.

300 g pitted dates, chopped

juice and finely grated zest
  of 2 oranges

1 teaspoon bicarb soda

2 eggs, lightly whisked

2 cups almond meal

¼ cup coconut flour

½ cup slivered almonds,
  toasted

3 teaspoons ground
  cinnamon

raspberries, to serve

Spiced Cream

2 × 400 ml cans coconut cream

1 tablespoon maple syrup

1 teaspoon mixed spice

1. Chill the cans of coconut cream for the Spiced Cream in the fridge overnight, so they'll be ready to go when you are.

2. To make the pudding, grease a 6-cup capacity ceramic pudding basin and line it with baking paper. Fill a large saucepan with water, put an upturned plate in it, and then put it over a medium heat. (The plate protects the pudding basin from the heat at the base of the pan.) Cover the pan and bring the water to a simmer.

3. Put the dates, orange zest and juice in a small saucepan over a medium heat and bring to a simmer. Simmer, stirring occasionally, for 3 minutes, or until the dates are slightly softened. Take the pan off the heat, then mash the date mixture and transfer it to a heat-proof bowl.

4. Add the remaining ingredients and stir until well combined. Spoon the mixture into the pudding basin and level the top. Cover the surface directly with a round piece of baking paper, then cover the basin with a sheet of baking paper and then a double sheet of foil. Secure the paper and foil around the lip of the pudding basin with cooking twine to form an airtight seal.

continued over page ⟶

5. Gently lower the pudding into the simmering pan of water and turn the heat down to low. Simmer very gently, topping up with boiling water as needed, for 4 hours, or until the pudding is cooked. You don't want it boiling dry, so make sure the water comes three-quarters of the way up the side of the pudding basin. When it's done, carefully lift the pudding out of the pan and let it stand, covered, for 20 minutes. While it stands, put a mixing bowl in the freezer to chill.

6. To make the spiced cream, take the chilled bowl from the freezer. Open the chilled cans of coconut cream, then spoon the thick layer of cream off the top and into the chilled bowl. You will need 1½ cups of this firm cream. (You can use the leftover coconut milk in your breakfast smoothies.) Add the maple syrup and mixed spice and whisk using an electric mixer until soft peaks form. Keep the cream chilled until ready to serve.

7. Take the paper and foil off the pudding and turn the pudding upright onto a serving plate. Top with raspberries, then serve warm with the spiced cream.

Summer Trifle

Serves 6

Nothing says summer in Australia like a trifle – it's the perfect dessert to share, and it looks gorgeous in a big glass bowl. Impress your friends with this paleo take on a classic indulgence.

blueberries, to serve

Jelly

250 g raspberries, plus extra
  to serve

2 tablespoons rice syrup

3 teaspoons powdered gelatine

Custard

6 egg yolks, at room temperature

¼ cup rice syrup

⅓ cup arrowroot

2 cups unsweetened almond
  milk

2 vanilla beans, seeds scraped

1 teaspoon powdered gelatine

1. To make the jelly, put the raspberries, rice syrup and 1½ cups of water in a small saucepan over a medium heat and bring to the boil. Boil, stirring occasionally, for 5 minutes, or until the raspberries have collapsed and the liquid has slightly reduced. Take the pan off the heat and let it stand for 5 minutes to cool slightly.

2. Pour the raspberry mixture into a food processor and blend until smooth, then push it through a sieve into a bowl. Discard the leftover seeds, then whisk the gelatine into the warm raspberry liquid until it's dissolved.

3. Pour the liquid into a deep, round, 6-cup capacity glass serving dish, then let it cool to room temperature. Put it in the fridge to chill for 2 hours, or until firm. (Don't put the hot bowl straight into the fridge, as it may shatter.) While the jelly sets, start on the custard.

4. To make the custard, whisk the egg yolks, rice syrup and arrowroot together until pale and creamy. Heat the almond milk with the vanilla seeds in a small saucepan over a low heat until it reaches boiling point, then slowly whisk the hot milk mixture into the yolk mixture until well combined and smooth.

continued over page →

Crumble

1 cup whole raw almonds, roasted

1 cup pepitas

1 cup pistachios, roasted

⅓ cup hemp seeds

5. Pour the milk and egg mixture into a clean saucepan and cook, stirring constantly, over a medium-low heat for 4 minutes, or until thick and smooth. Take the pan off the heat and whisk in the gelatine until it dissolves and is well combined and smooth. Strain into a heat-proof bowl and cover the surface directly with cling film to prevent a skin forming, then let it cool to room temperature. While it cools, start on the crumble.

6. To make the crumble, put all the ingredients in a food processor and process until coarse crumbs form. Spoon half the crumb mixture over the surface of the firmly set raspberry jelly, then set aside the rest.

7. Spoon the custard over the crumb layer in the dish. Sprinkle with the remaining crumb mixture and top with extra raspberries and blueberries before serving.

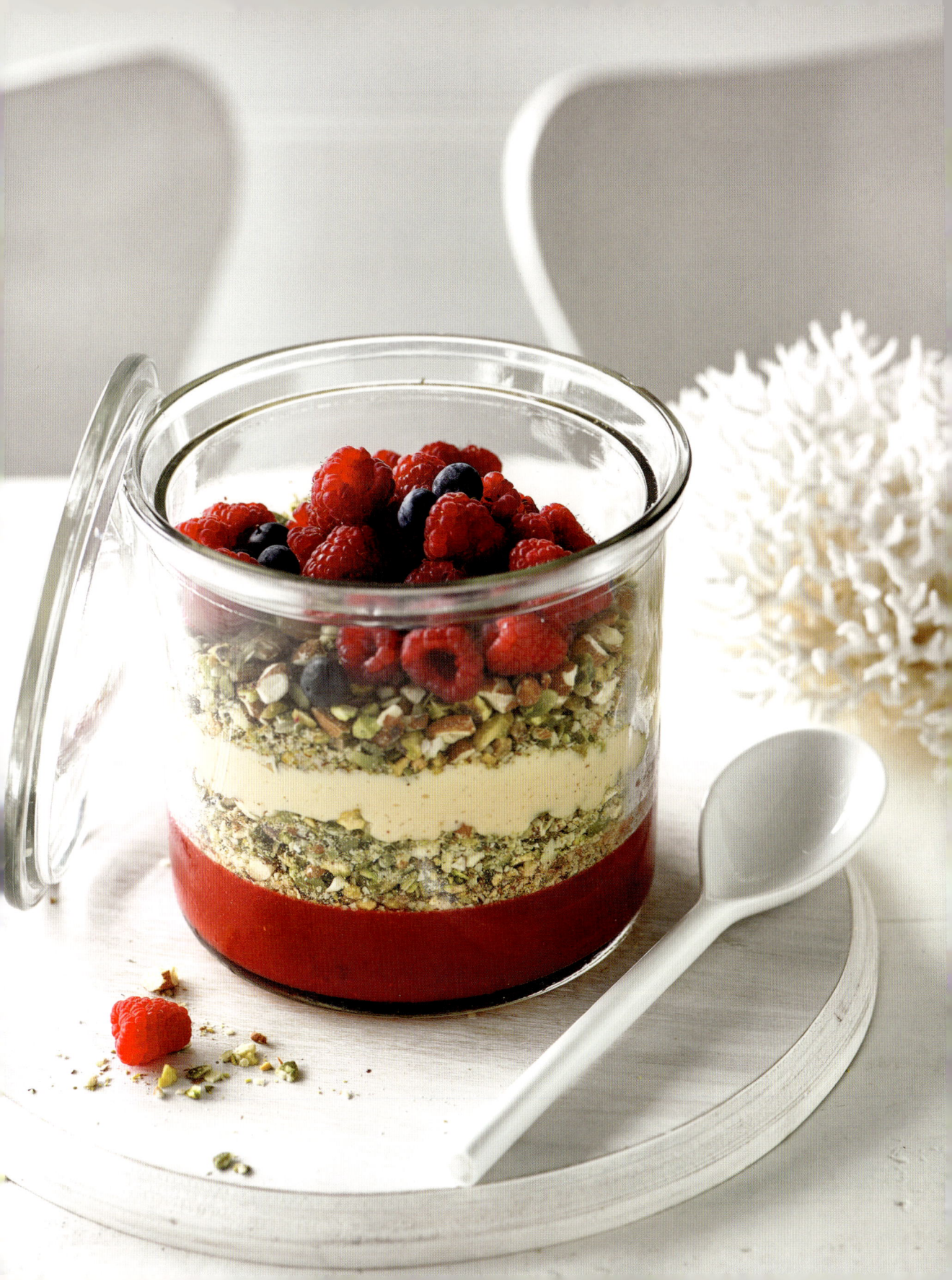

Festive Panforte

Serves 16

This makes a great Christmas cake alternative – though we'd eat it all year round. Full of great spices, it has all the festive joy you are craving.

¼ cup coconut flour

3 teaspoons mixed spice

½ cup raw cacao powder

1 cup raw sliced almonds, toasted

1 cup hazelnuts, toasted, skins rubbed off, chopped

250 g pitted dates, chopped

1 tablespoon finely grated orange zest

1 tablespoon finely grated lemon zest

⅓ cup maple syrup

⅔ cup melted coconut oil, cooled but runny

desiccated coconut, to sprinkle

1. Grease a 22 cm round springform cake tin and line it with baking paper.
2. Put all the ingredients together in a large bowl and stir until well combined. The mixture should feel firm and slightly sticky. Spoon it into the cake tin and level the top by pressing it down firmly with the palm of your hand. (If your hand is damp, the mixture won't stick to it.) Chill for 1 hour, or until firm.
3. Take the panforte out of the fridge, then sprinkle the top with coconut. Release the side of the cake tin and transfer the panforte to a serving plate. Let it stand for 10 minutes before slicing into wedges and serving.

TIP: Keep panforte chilled so that it stays firm. Panforte will keep in an airtight container in the fridge for up to 1 month.

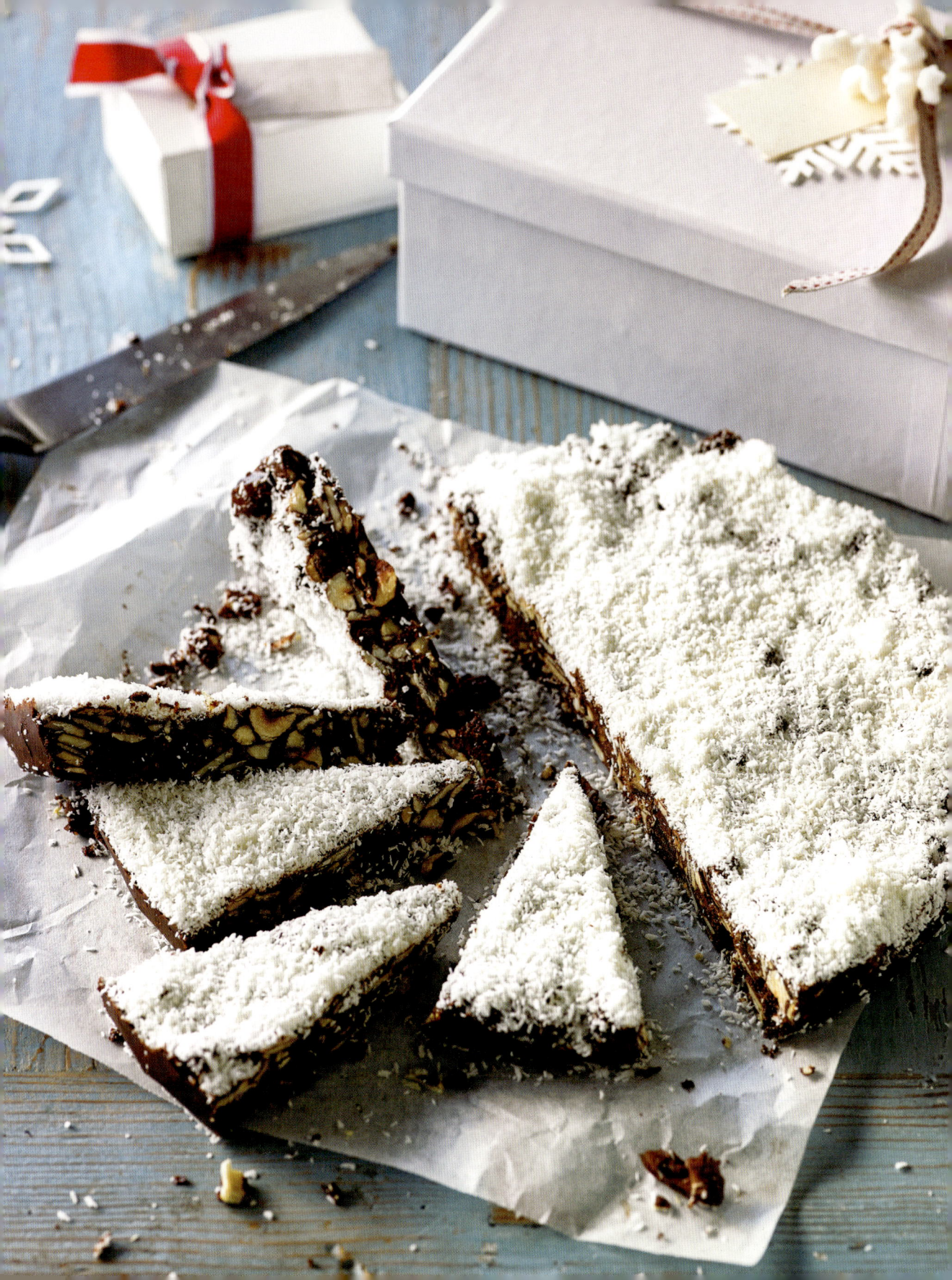

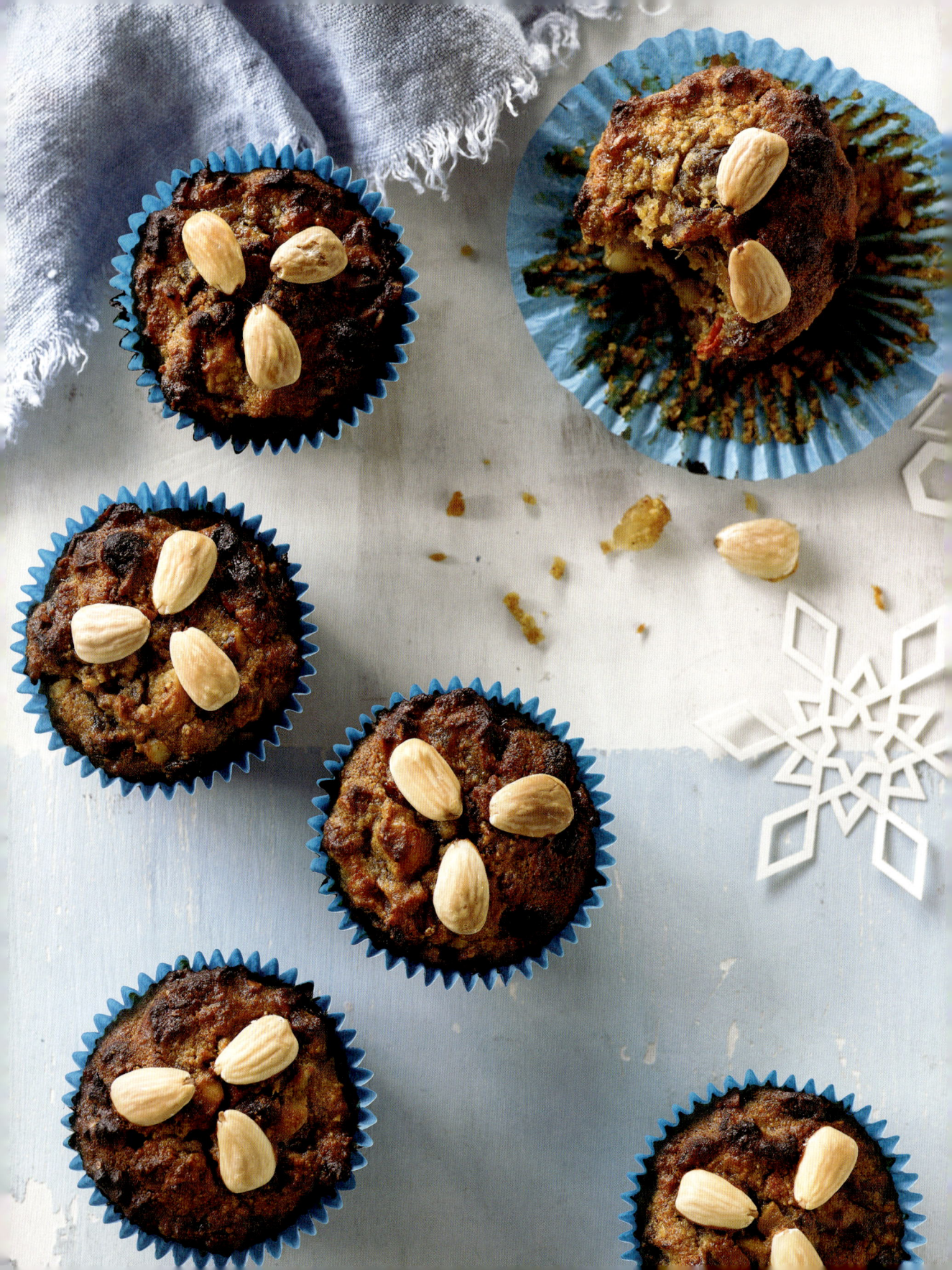

Individual Christmas Cakes

Makes 12

You can't escape the scent of Christmas cakes throughout December while you're shopping, so head home and make these great-looking and much healthier individual serves for the big day.

250 g pitted dates, chopped

¾ cup dried goji berries

juice and finely grated zest of 1 orange

⅓ cup brandy

100 g butter, melted and cooled

½ cup maple syrup

1 cup brazil nuts, finely chopped and toasted

1 cup macadamias, finely chopped and toasted

2 teaspoons mixed spice

4 eggs, at room temperature, lightly whisked

½ cup almond meal

¼ cup coconut flour

36 whole blanched almonds

1. Preheat your oven to 180°C and line a 12-hole muffin pan with paper patty cases.
2. Put the dates, goji berries, orange juice and zest, and brandy in a small saucepan over a medium heat and bring to the boil. Boil for 2 minutes, or until the brandy has reduced by half and the dates have slightly softened. Transfer to a large, heat-proof bowl and set aside for a few minutes to cool slightly.
3. Add all the remaining ingredients to the date mixture in the bowl and mix well to combine. Spoon evenly into the patty cases. (The mixture will sit high in the patty cases.) Top each with 3 almonds, then bake for 25 minutes, or until golden. When they're cooked, a skewer inserted in the centre should come out clean. Let the cakes cool in the pan for 5 minutes, then turn them out onto a wire rack. Serve warm or at room temperature.

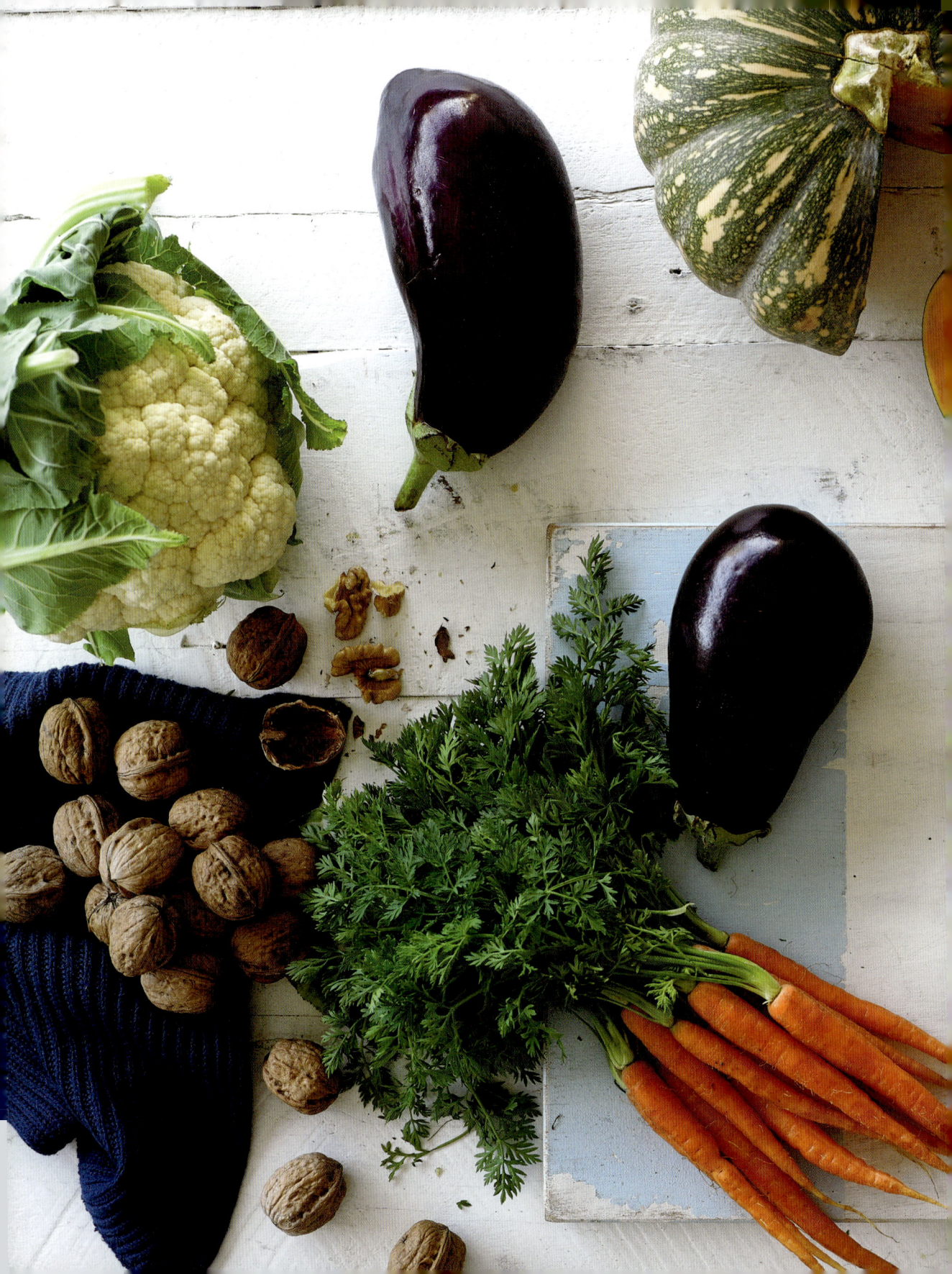

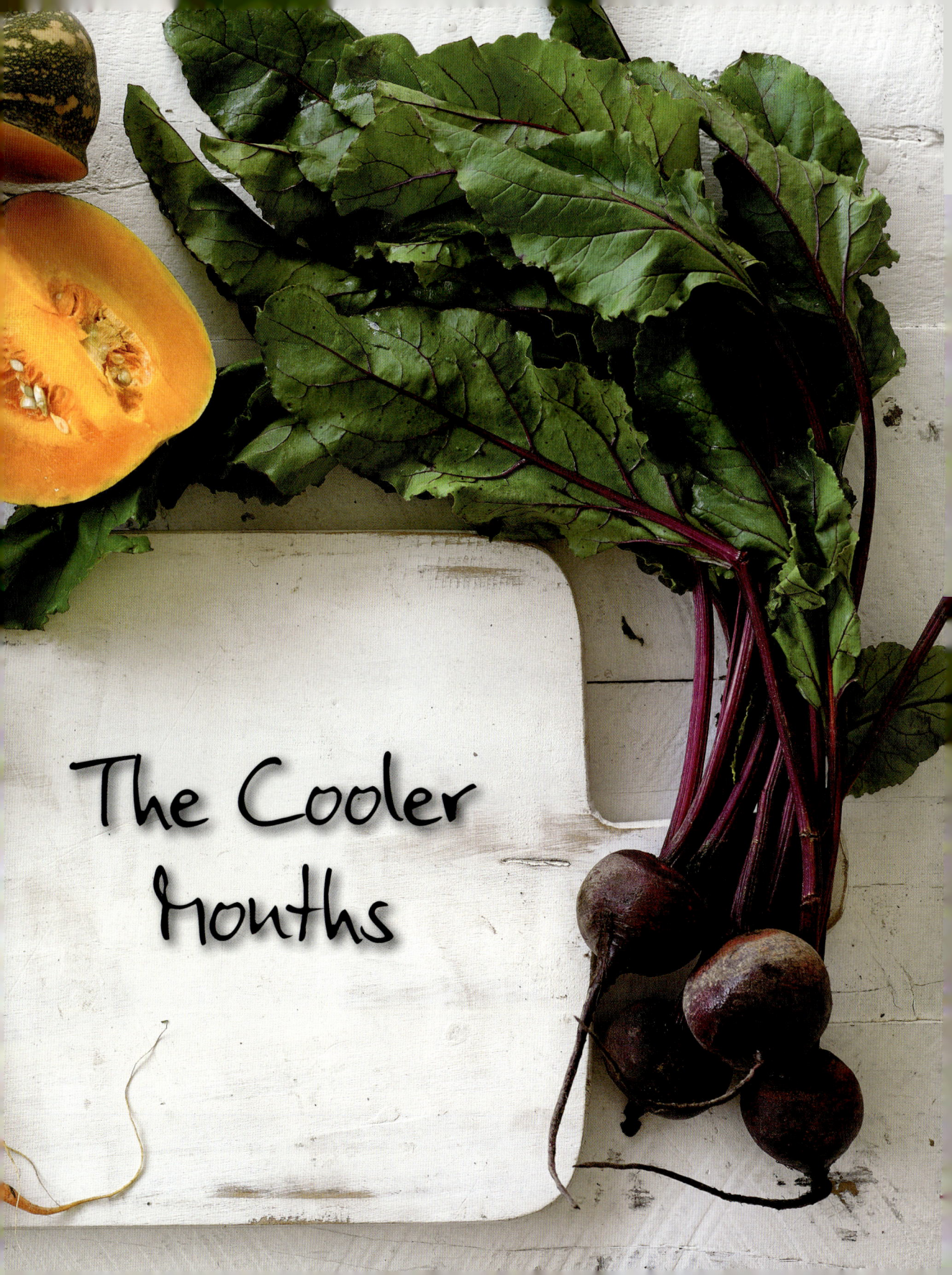

The Cooler Months

Braised Lamb Necks 63

Poached Chicken in Chicken Broth 64

Mum's Meatloaf 67

Wild Mushroom Soup 68

Roast Pork with Caraway Seeds 71

Twelve-Hour Roasted Lamb Shoulder 72

Chicken Zoodle Soup 75

Pork-and-Fennel-Stuffed Jalapeños 76

Caponata-Stuffed Pork Belly 79

Beef Short Ribs with Turmeric Cauli Rice 80

Rabbit Stroganoff 83

Quail Scotch Eggs 84

Pork and Pistachio Terrine 87

Coconut Berry Tartlets   88
Hazelnut Butter Cups   91
Chilled Lemon Curd Creams   92
Sweet Pumpkin Pie   95
Chargrilled Coconut Waffles   96
Cacao Chip Cookies   99
Self-Saucing Cacao Pudding   100
Apple Crumble Slice   103
Raspberry Coconut Truffles   104
Hot Cross Buns   107
Easter Eggs   108
Tess's Spiced Dream Cake   111

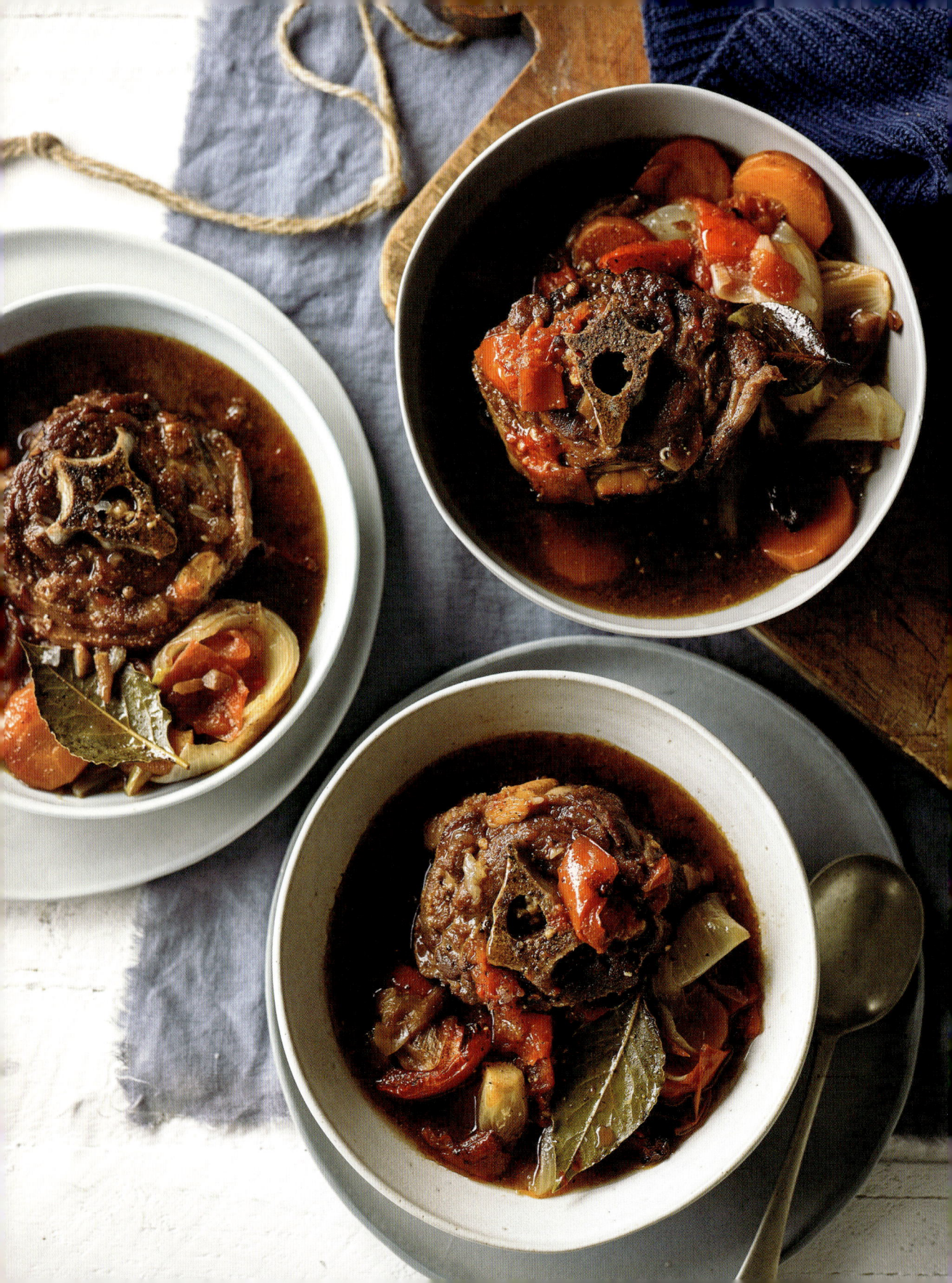

Braised Lamb Necks

Serves 3

Scott says: 'Much of my inspiration has come from my upbringing in the UK. My folks ran pubs in and around London, where full-bodied, hearty braised dishes were often the cornerstone of the menu. This recipe is a throwback to those days.'

2 tablespoons coconut oil

2 lamb necks, each cut into
  3 rounds (ask your butcher to
  do this)

4 garlic cloves, roughly chopped

2 carrots, sliced

1 large leek, halved crosswise,
  then each piece halved
  lengthwise

6 eschalots, peeled

1 brown onion, peeled and
  quartered

splash of red wine

1 kg tomatoes, roughly chopped

4 cups beef or chicken stock

1 teaspoon coriander seeds

1 teaspoon sweet paprika

2 bay leaves

sea salt and ground black pepper

1. Preheat your oven to 170° C.

2. Heat 1 tablespoon of the coconut oil in a frying pan. Once it's hot, drop in the lamb neck rounds. You may have to do this in batches. When the necks are completely browned and sealed, take them off the heat. Set the necks aside in a casserole dish or deep baking dish.

3. Add more oil to the frying pan, if you need it, then add the garlic and veggies and fry until golden brown.

4. Transfer the veggies to the casserole dish with the meat and then, while the pan is still hot, deglaze it with the red wine, scraping up all the delicious bits stuck on the bottom. Pour the liquid over the meat and veggies.

5. Add the tomatoes, stock, coriander seeds, paprika, bay leaves, salt and pepper to the casserole dish, then chuck it in the oven, uncovered, for around 2½ hours. The lamb is done when the meat falls away from the bone. Take it out of the oven and let it stand for 10 minutes before serving.

Poached Chicken in Chicken Broth

Serves 2

This recipe oozes goodness – broth is a major promoter of gut health. The added chicken thighs make it a hearty winter warmer.

4 cups easy chicken broth
(see recipe on page 133)

150 g chicken thigh meat,
chopped

1 baby fennel bulb, thinly sliced

1 carrot, thinly sliced

2 eschalots, finely chopped

1 cup roughly chopped kale

1 teaspoon chilli powder
(optional)

1 teaspoon butter (optional)

1. Put the broth in a large saucepan over a medium-high heat and bring to a simmer. Add the chicken, fennel, carrot and eschalots and cook for 5 minutes.
2. Add the kale and cook for a further 5 minutes.
3. Take the pan off the heat and add the chilli and butter (if using) before serving.

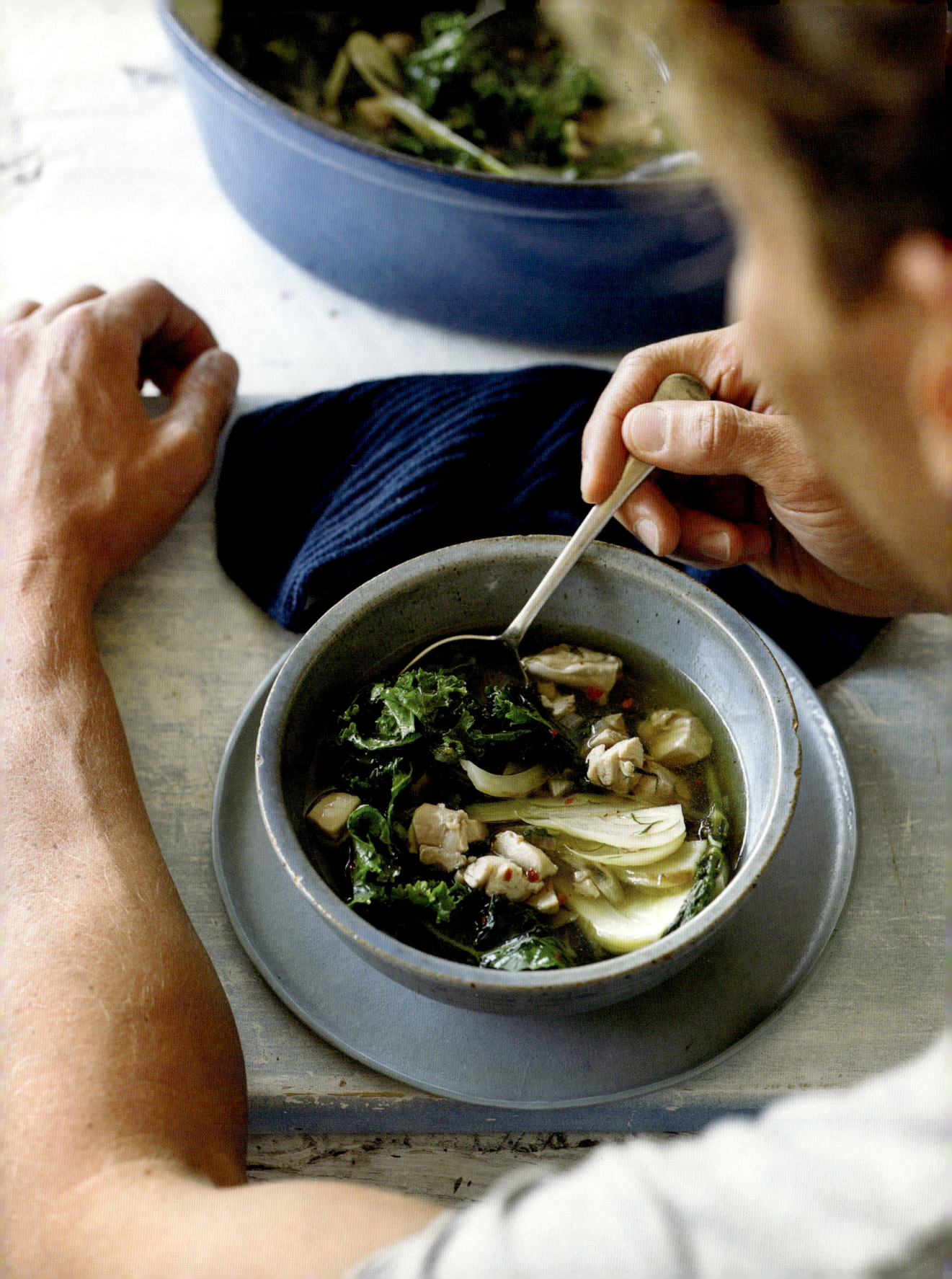

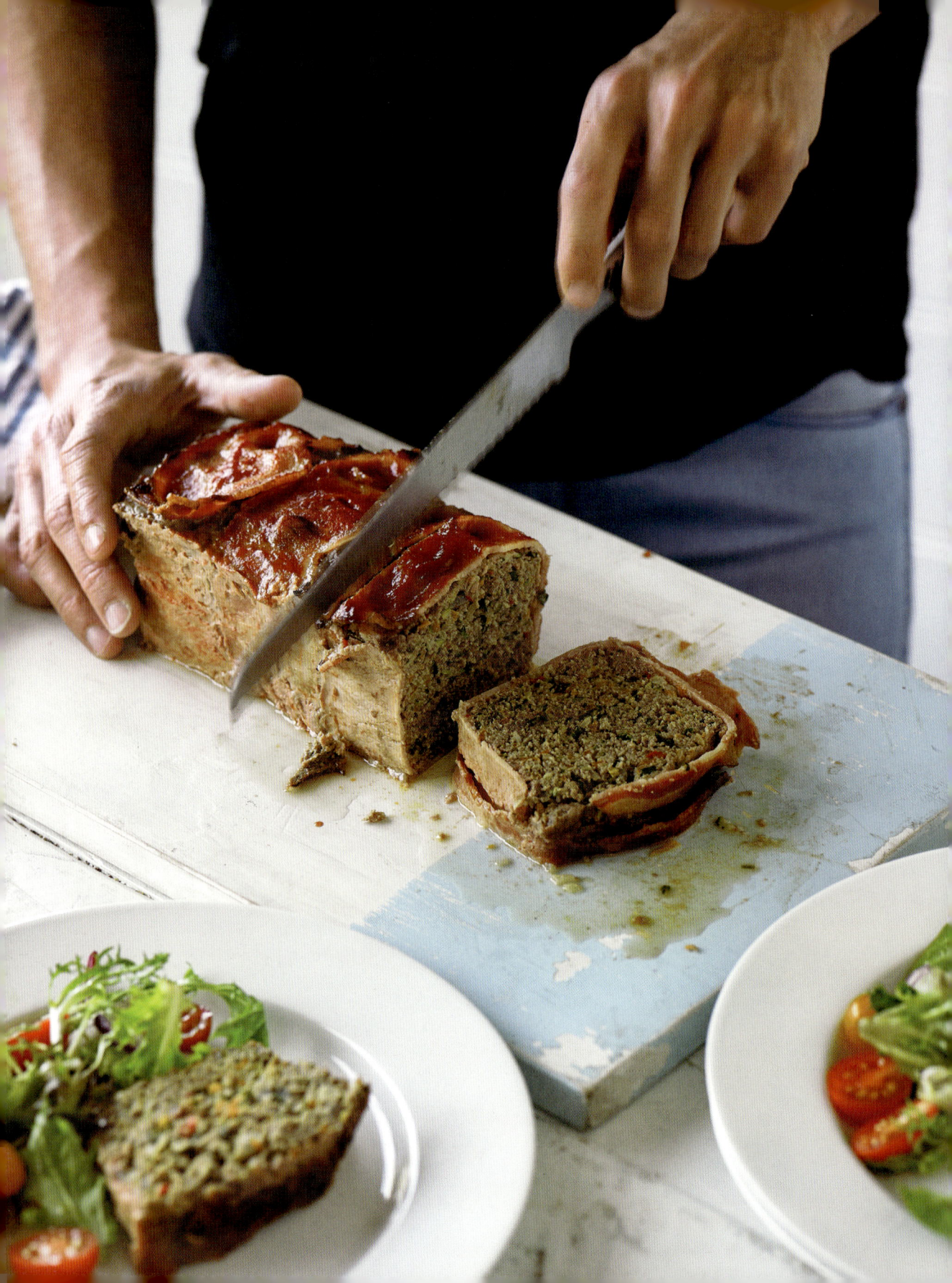

Mum's Meatloaf

Serves 6-8

Luke says: 'This recipe reminds me of my childhood. My mum used to make the most amazing meatloaf, and this is a paleofied version of it. I hope you enjoy it!'

4 large rashers rindless bacon

4 tablespoons coconut oil

2 red onions, finely diced

1 carrot, grated

2 stalks celery, finely chopped

2 garlic cloves, crushed

1 long red chilli, chopped
(optional)

2 zucchini, grated

750 g beef mince

4 tablespoons almond meal

4 tablespoons flat-leaf parsley,
roughly chopped

2 eggs, lightly whisked

1 teaspoon ground cumin

1 tablespoon sea salt

2 teaspoons ground black
pepper

⅓ cup coconut milk

⅓ cup tomato passata

1 tablespoon honey

1 tablespoon apple cider vinegar

1. Preheat your oven to 180°C and line a large loaf tin with baking paper, letting the paper extend a few centimetres above the sides.

2. Line the base and long sides of the prepared tin crosswise with the bacon, allowing lengths to overhang, as you will fold these over later.

3. Put 2 tablespoons of the coconut oil in a frying pan crosswise over a medium heat. When it's hot, add the onions, carrot and celery and cook for 5 minutes, or until softened, then add the garlic, chilli and zucchini and cook for a further 3 minutes. Drain off any liquid and set the veggies aside to cool completely.

4. Put the mince, almond meal, parsley, cooked veggies, eggs, cumin, salt, pepper and coconut milk in a bowl with the remaining 2 tablespoons of coconut oil and mix until well combined.

5. Pack the meat mixture into the lined loaf tin, then fold the overhanging bacon rashers over the top. Put the meatloaf on a baking tray and pop it into the oven to bake, setting a timer to go off after 25 minutes.

6. Meanwhile, mix the tomato passata, honey and vinegar in a small bowl. When the timer goes off, take the meatloaf out of the oven and baste the top with the tomato mixture. Return it to the oven and continue cooking for a further 25 minutes, or until cooked through.

7. Let the meatloaf rest for 10 minutes before turning it out of the tin.

Wild Mushroom Soup

Serves 4

Mushrooms are so tasty that their health benefits are often overlooked. Chaga mushrooms, for example, have anti-inflammatory properties, boosting the immune system and helping to fight cancer. The fact that they taste great is a bonus! Other varieties that work well in this recipe are porcini, chanterelle, portobello and good old field mushrooms.

1 tablespoon butter or ghee

2 eschalots, finely chopped

handful thyme leaves, roughly chopped

2 sage leaves, shredded

500 g mixed mushrooms, trimmed, thickly sliced

2 cups easy chicken broth (see recipe on page 133)

2 cups coconut cream

1. Melt the butter in a saucepan over a high heat. When it begins to froth, add the eschalots, thyme and sage, and cook for 1 minute, or until the eschalots start to soften.

2. Add the mushrooms and cook for 6–8 minutes, or until browned and just starting to soften, then add the stock and simmer, uncovered, for 15–20 minutes. Add the coconut cream and stir gently for 2–3 minutes, then take the pan off the heat. Serve the soup in bowls or cups.

NOTE: We use a combination of shiitake, enoki, shimeji, woodear, oyster and field mushrooms.

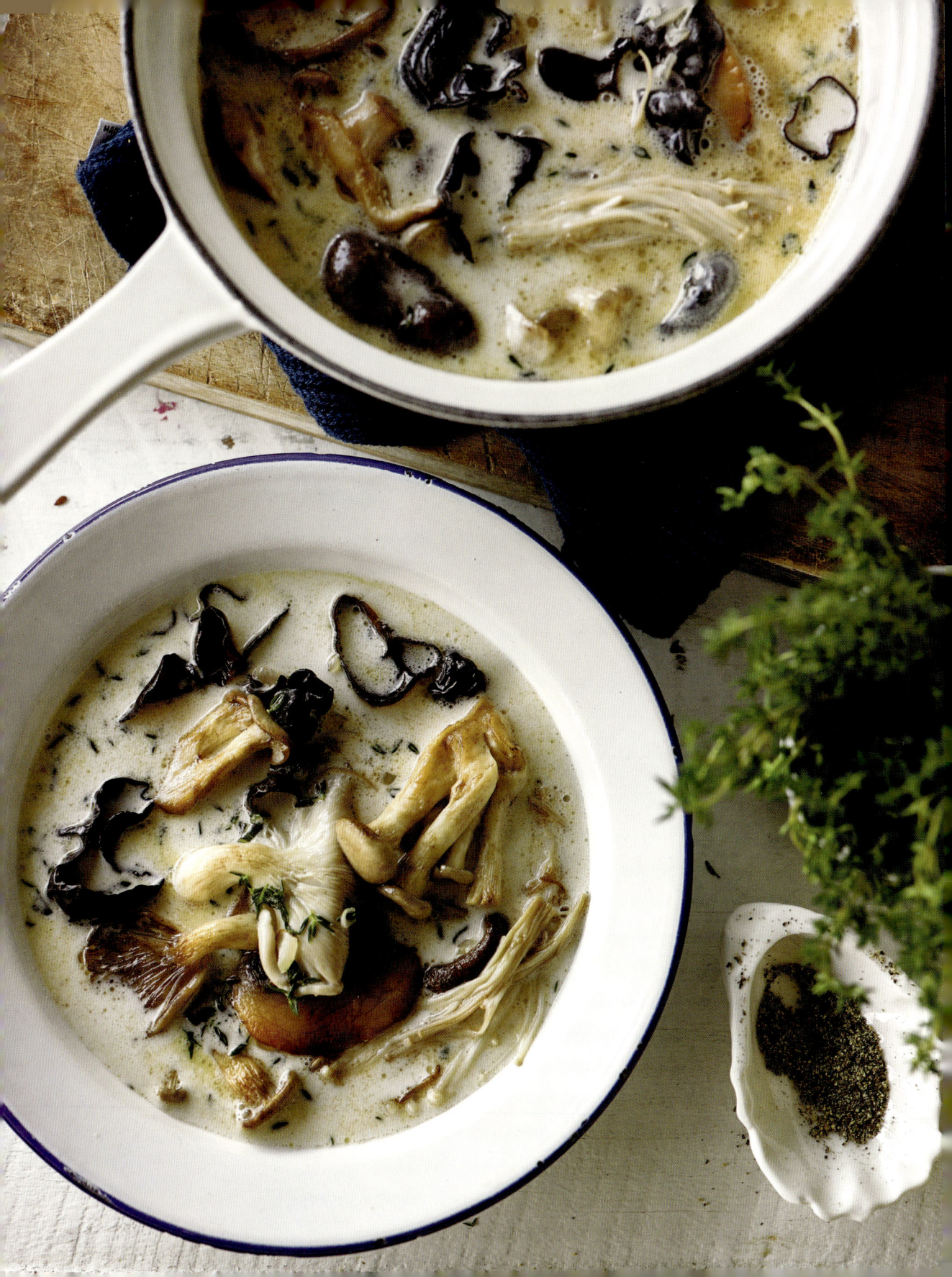

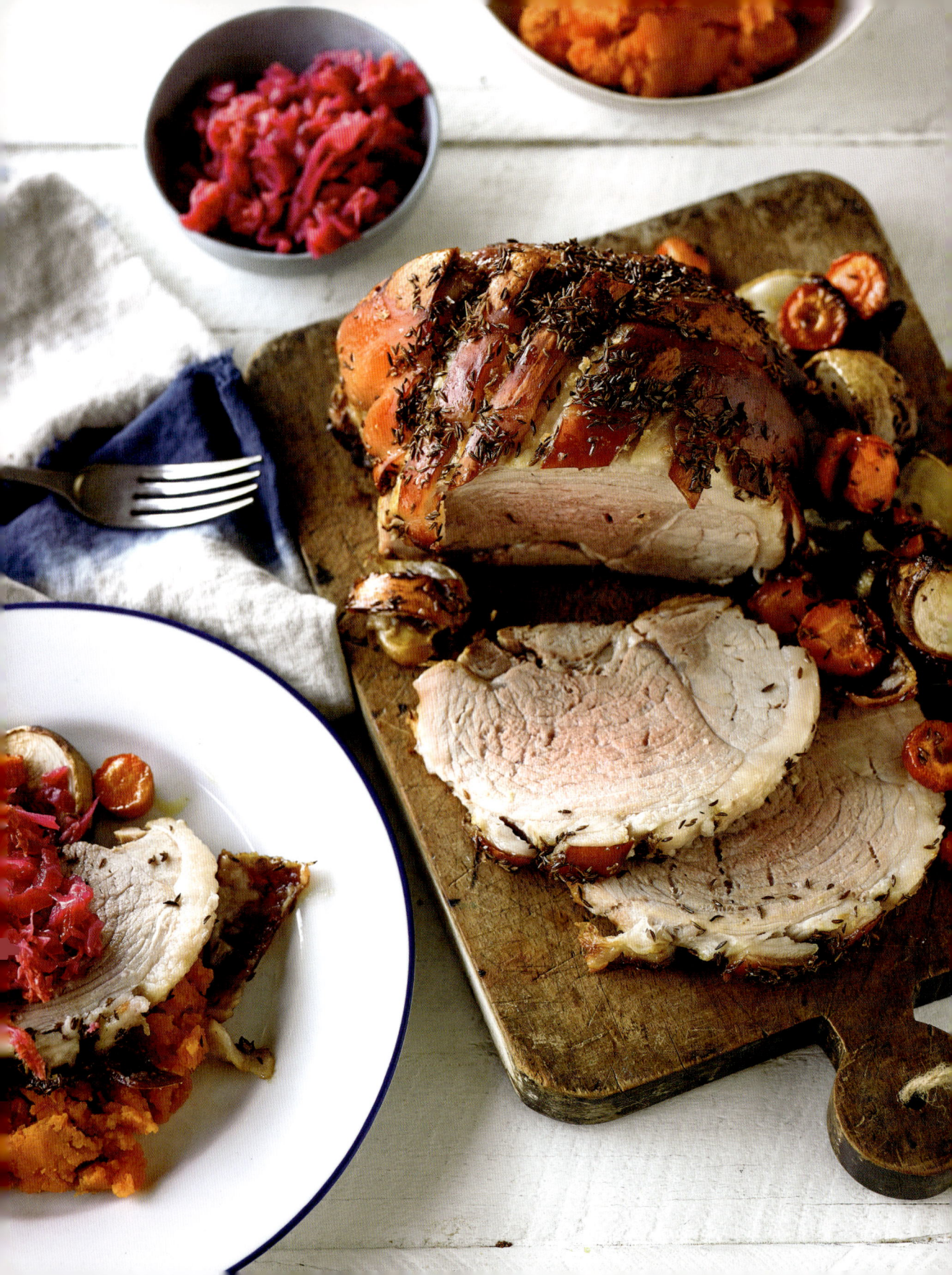

Roast Pork with Caraway Seeds

Serves 4

What's better than crispy-skin pork? This succulent dish always delivers and it's super-easy too. It's great served with sweet potato mash, or sauerkraut, or both.

2 kg boned pork loin roast, trussed, rind scored

2 brown onions, thinly sliced

2 garlic cloves, thinly sliced

1 tablespoon coconut oil

1 turnip, roughly chopped

2 carrots, roughly chopped

sea salt

juice of 1 lemon

1 tablespoon cumin seeds

2 tablespoons caraway seeds

sauerkraut (see recipe on page 118)

1. To ensure the pork rind crisps up nicely, pop the pork loin in the fridge for 1 hour. Remove and pat dry with paper towel.

2. Preheat your oven to 220°C.

3. Put the onions and garlic in a baking dish and pop the pork on top.

4. Combine the coconut oil and chopped veggies in a bowl, season them with salt and then arrange them around the pork.

5. Pour the lemon juice on the rind, then sprinkle it with salt and the cumin seeds and caraway seeds. Rub the spices into the rind, then put the pork in the oven for 20 minutes before turning the heat down. Let it roast another 1½–2 hours, or until cooked to your liking. Take the pork out of the oven and let it rest for 20 minutes before carving. Serve with sauerkraut or some creamy sweet potato mash. Enjoy!

Twelve-Hour Roasted Lamb Shoulder

Serves 6

This sounds like hard work, but it's the easiest crowd-pleasing dish around – simply prepare your lamb and have it in its baking dish the night before, then pop it in the oven first thing in the morning and forget all about it until dinnertime. All you have to do then is toss together a simple green salad and serve it up.

2 tablespoons coconut oil

50 g butter

2 red onions, sliced into rounds

core and fronds of 2 fennel bulbs, sliced

sea salt and ground black pepper

2 x 750 g boned lamb shoulders

3 sprigs rosemary

500 g large cherry tomatoes, halved

2 garlic bulbs, outer dry skin rubbed away (leave whole)

lemon wedges, to serve

green salad, to serve

1. If you're going to put the lamb on to cook straightaway, preheat your oven to 110°C. If you're not going to cook it until the next day, just do steps 2 and 3, then leave the baking dish in the fridge overnight and preheat the oven as soon as you get up in the morning.

2. Melt the coconut oil and butter together in a large saucepan over a medium heat. When the pan is hot, add the onions and fennel. Cook, stirring, for 10 minutes, or until the veggies are very soft and starting to turn golden brown. Take the pan off the heat and let the veggies cool, then season them with salt and pepper.

3. Put half the onion mixture in a large, heavy baking dish. Rest the lamb on top and spoon the remaining onion mixture over it. Add the rosemary, tomatoes and garlic to the dish, then season with salt and pepper. Cover the dish with baking paper and then a double sheet of foil.

4. Put the lamb into the oven to roast for 12 hours, or until the meat falls easily off the bone when tested with a fork. Let it rest in the dish, covered, for 10 minutes, then serve it straight to the table with lemon wedges and a green salad on the side.

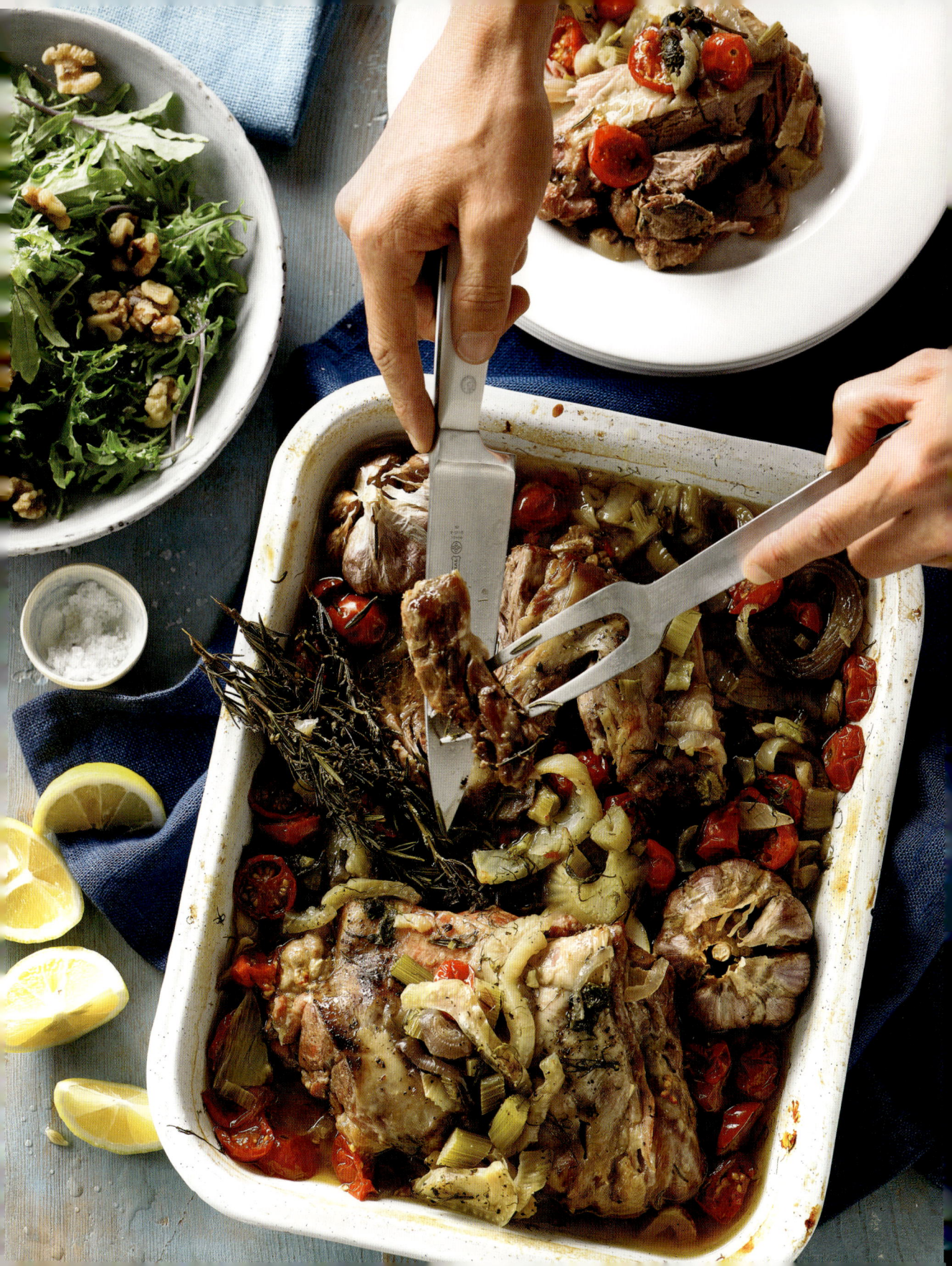

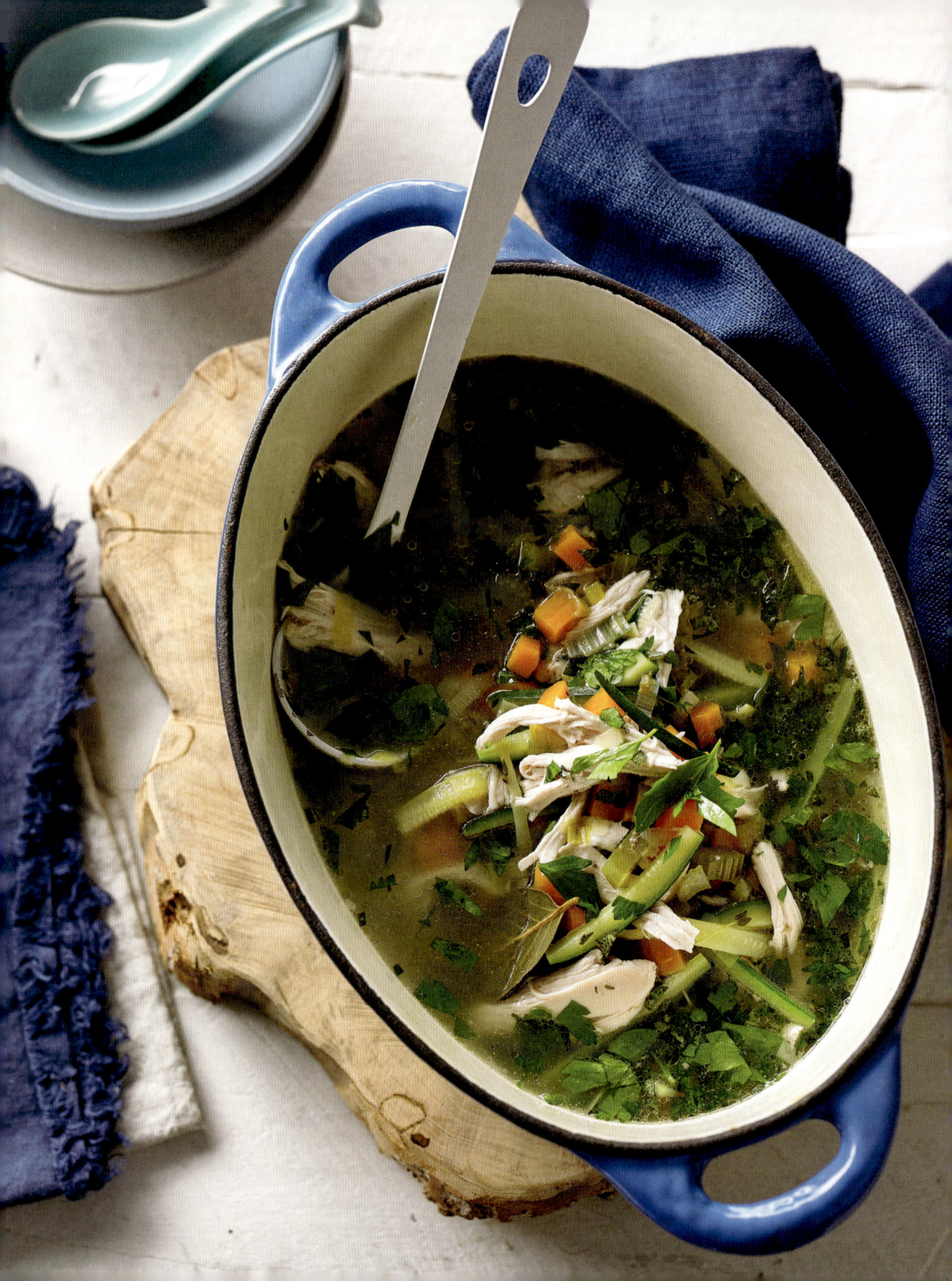

Chicken Zoodle Soup

Serves 6

Whenever you're feeling a little under the weather, there's nothing like the restorative powers of a delicious chicken soup. This one has zoodles – zucchini noodles – in place of the usual starchy wheat noodles. It's an easy and very warming dish that will have you feeling better from the first sip!

1.5 kg whole chicken

1 large leek, white part only, sliced

2 carrots, chopped

3 stalks celery, chopped

2 dried bay leaves

2 tablespoons thyme leaves

3 litres filtered water

2 zucchini

1 tablespoon finely chopped sage

½ cup chopped flat-leaf parsley

1. Rinse the chicken inside and out under cold running water, then put it in a large saucepan, breast side down. Add the leek, carrots, celery, bay leaves and thyme. Season, then add the water.

2. Put the pan over a high heat and bring to the boil, then turn the heat down to low and let it simmer, partially covered, for 1½ hours, or until the chicken is cooked. Use a large slotted spoon to skim away any impurities or froth that rise to the surface as it simmers.

3. Take the pan off the heat, then carefully lift the chicken out and put it in a large, heat-proof bowl. Discard all the skin and bones, then shred the meat.

4. Cut the zucchini into matchsticks, to resemble noodles, and add them to the soup in the pan. Put the pan back on the stove over a medium heat and let it simmer for 4 minutes, or until the zoodles are just tender.

5. Discard the bay leaves, then stir the chicken meat, sage and parsley through the soup. Season to taste before serving.

Pork-and-Fennel-Stuffed Jalapeños

Makes 24

Fresh jalapeños make the perfect spicy-but-sweet home for this delicious pork and fennel stuffing – a great little snack to have when it's a bit cooler out.

100 g pork mince

2 teaspoons fennel seeds

⅓ cup coarsely grated carrot

2 spring onions, thinly sliced

sea salt and ground black pepper

12 large fresh green jalapeños, halved lengthwise, seeds removed

12 slices prosciutto, halved crosswise

lemon wedges, to serve

1. Preheat your oven to 200°C and line a large baking tray with baking paper.
2. Put the mince, fennel seeds, carrot and spring onions in a bowl and mix well to combine, then season to taste.
3. Divide the pork mixture between the halved jalapeños and press it down firmly. Wrap a piece of prosciutto around each one, then put them on the tray.
4. Bake in the oven for 25 minutes, or until the pork filling is cooked and the jalapeños are golden. Serve warm with lemon wedges.

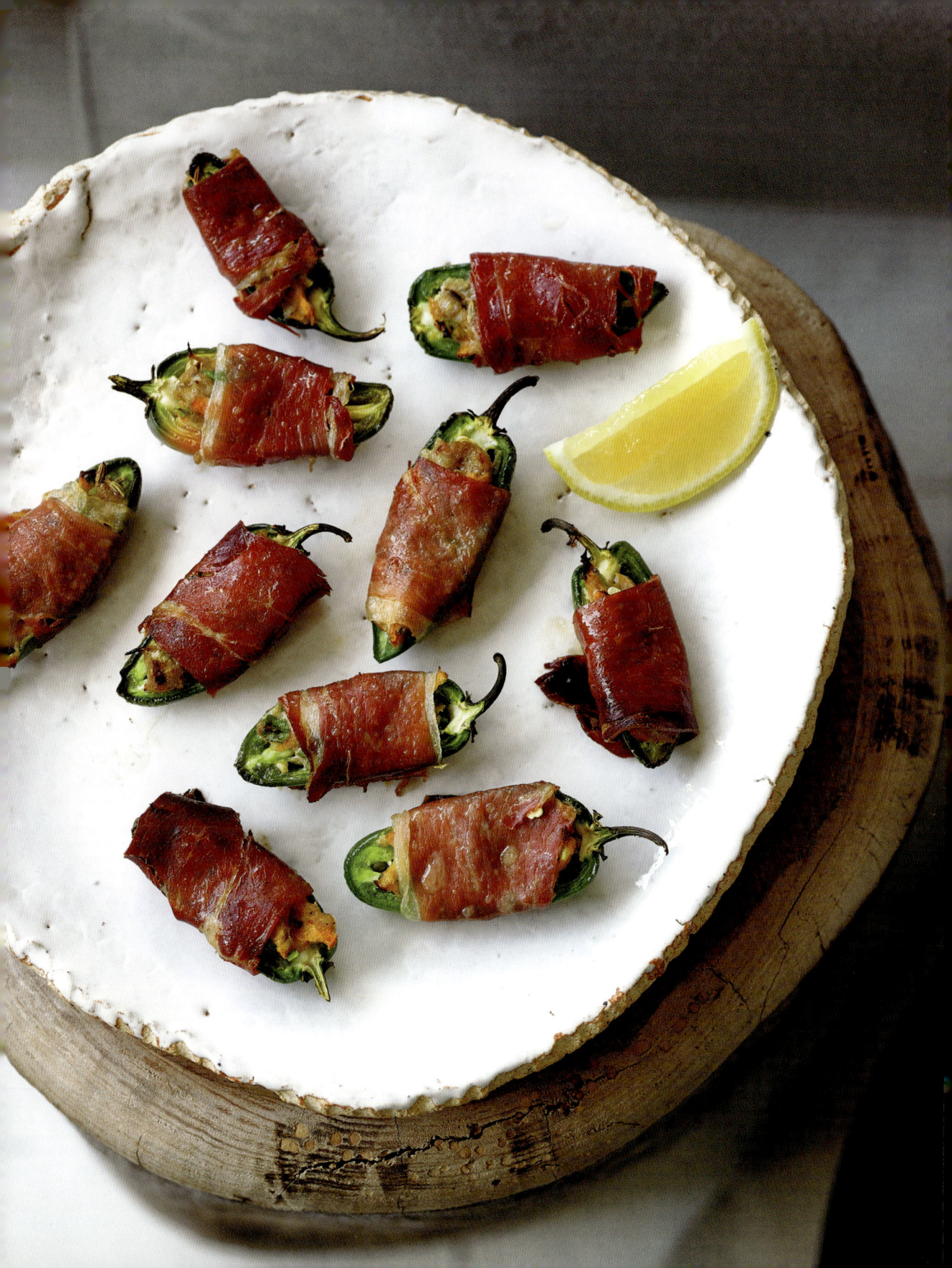

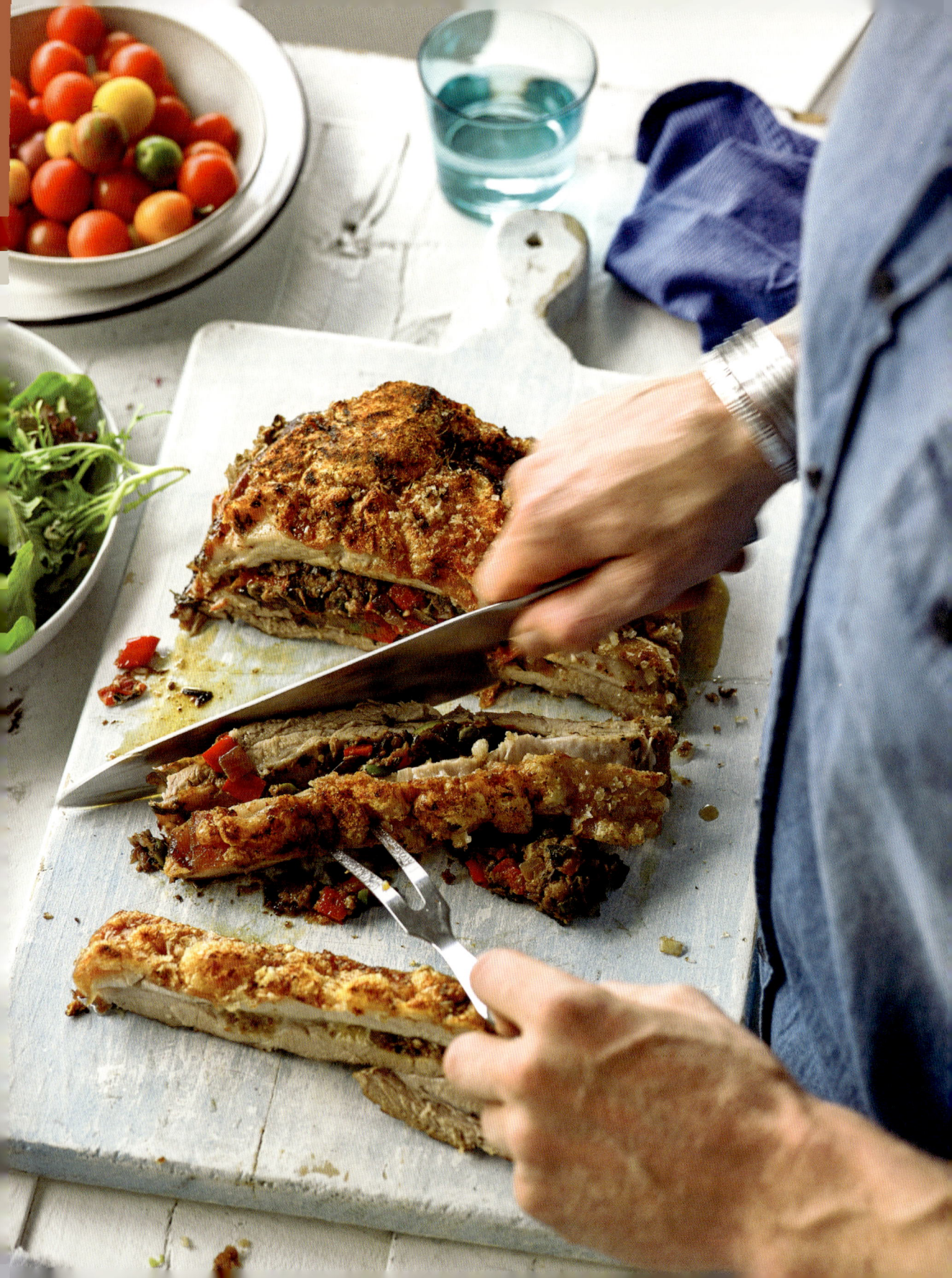

Caponata-Stuffed Pork Belly

Serves 6

We love pork belly no matter how it's cooked, but this mix of fresh Italian flavours and delicious veggies is one of our favourites.

1.2 kg pork belly, rind on and scored

1 tablespoon sea salt

green salad, to serve

Caponata

2 tablespoons coconut oil

1 small eggplant, chopped

1 small red onion, chopped

1 small red capsicum, chopped

150 g cherry tomatoes, quartered

1 tablespoon baby capers

6 large green Sicilian olives, pitted and chopped

2 garlic cloves, crushed

⅓ cup chopped basil

⅓ cup chopped flat-leaf parsley

freshly ground black pepper

1. Preheat your oven to 220°C.

2. To make the caponata, put the coconut oil in a large frying pan over a medium heat. When it's hot, add the eggplant and onion. Cook, stirring occasionally, for 5 minutes. Add the capsicum and tomatoes and cook, stirring occasionally, for 10 minutes, or until all the veggies have collapsed and are very tender. Take the pan off the heat and stir through the capers, olives, garlic, basil and parsley. Season with freshly ground black pepper, then set aside to cool.

3. Using a large sharp knife, make a horizontal incision through the centre of the pork meat to form a pocket, making sure not to cut all the way through to the sides. Fill the pocket with the cooled caponata mixture and secure the ends with toothpicks.

4. Put the pork on a greased wire rack over a large baking tray. Sprinkle sea salt over the rind, pushing it into the scored flesh.

5. Bake in the oven for 30 minutes, then turn the heat down to 180°C and cook for another hour, or until the pork is very tender and the rind is crisp and golden. Let it stand for 10 minutes, then slice crosswise. Serve with salad.

Beef Short Ribs with Turmeric Cauli Rice

Serves 6

Ribs are an affordable, full-flavoured cut of meat. Cooked long and low, the meat literally falls off the bone and melts in your mouth. This is one to try on the weekend, when you can take things slow.

6 short beef ribs

3 teaspoons aniseed seeds

2 teaspoons dried chilli flakes

1 tablespoon honey

2 tablespoons coconut oil

1 tablespoon beef tallow

sea salt and ground black pepper

coriander sprigs, to serve

Cauli Rice

¼ head cauliflower

1 tablespoon butter

½ teaspoon ground cumin

1 teaspoon ground turmeric

1. To prepare the ribs, preheat your oven to 120°C and line a roasting pan with foil, letting the foil extend a few centimetres above the sides.
2. Combine all the ingredients in a bowl, ensuring the meat is thoroughly coated in the spices, honey, seasoning and coconut oil, then empty the bowl into the pan and spread the ribs out evenly.
3. Lay another sheet of foil over the top of the ribs, tucking it in beneath them. Fold the first sheet of foil in over the sides to seal in the oil, then pop the tray in the oven for 6–8 hours.
4. To make the cauli rice, roughly chop up the cauli and chuck it in a blender, then process until it has a similar texture to rice. Melt the butter in a frying pan over a high heat, then throw in the cauli. Add the cumin and turmeric and fry for 4–5 minutes, season to taste, and cook for another 30 seconds before taking it off the heat. Sit the ribs on the rice, top with coriander sprigs and tuck in!

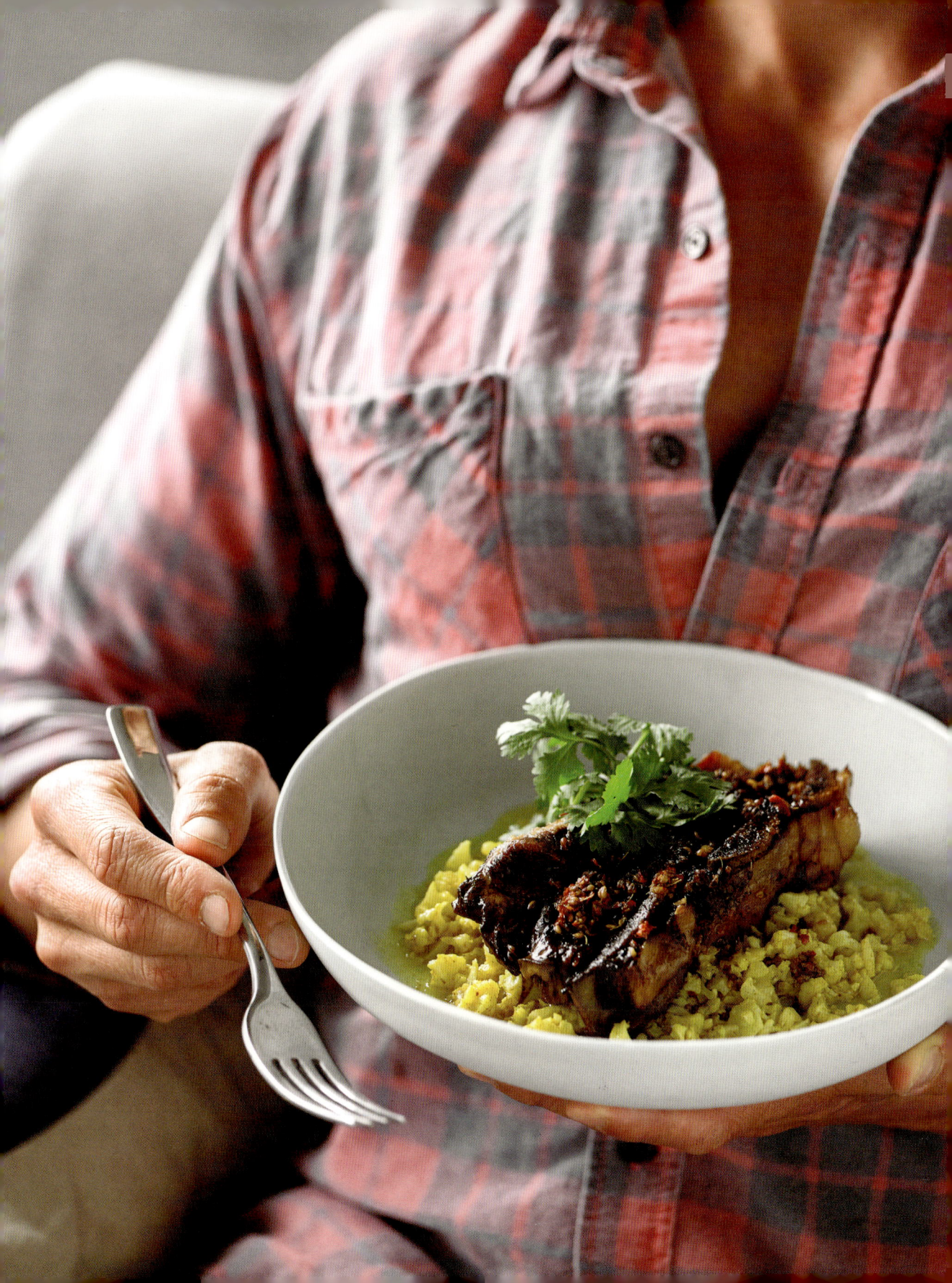

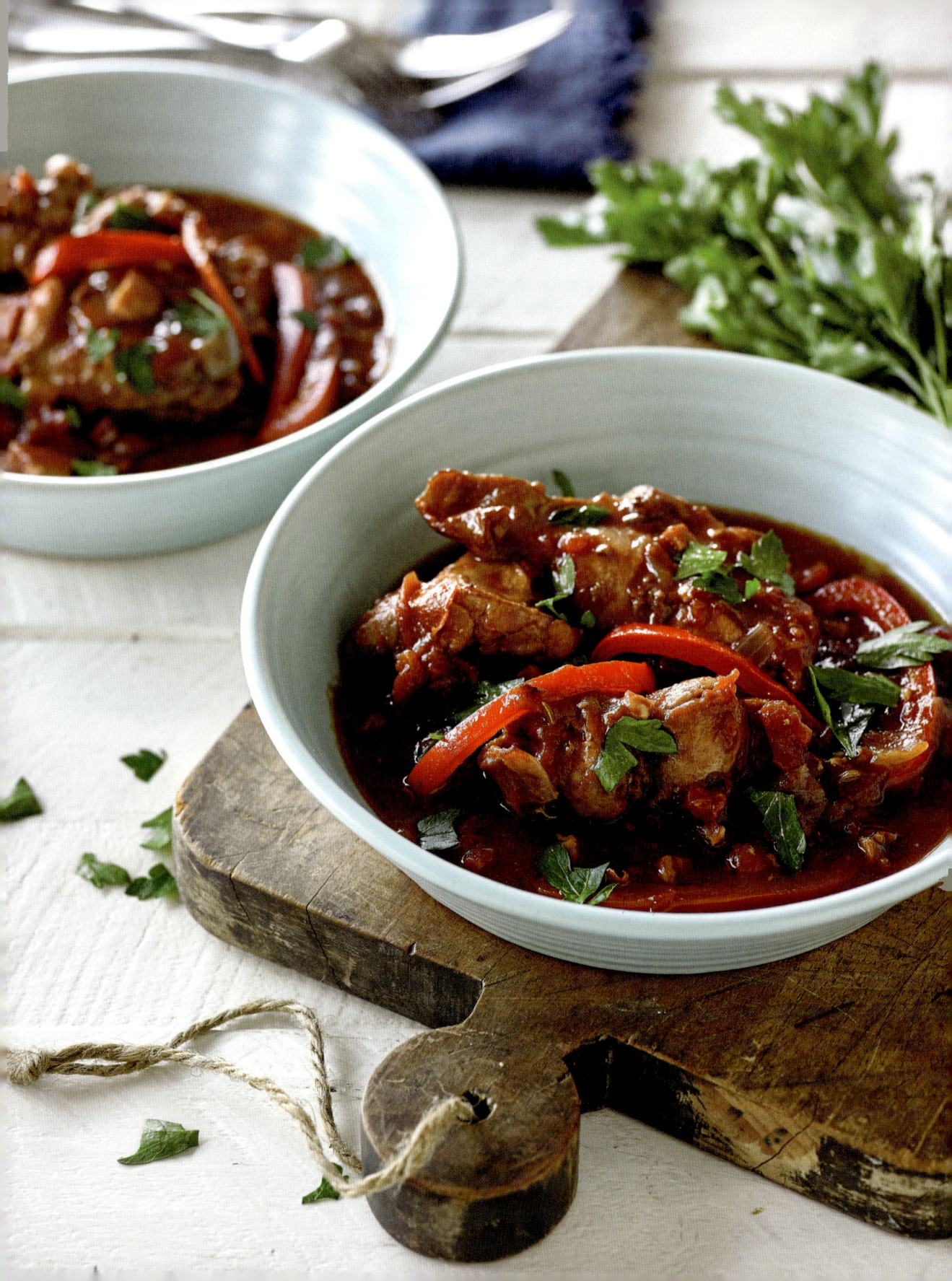

Rabbit Stroganoff

Serves 4-6

Rabbit and other game meats are delicious and full of flavour. They taste different from the standard cuts of beef and lamb you get from the butcher, and there is evidence to suggest they are easier for your body to digest. This twist on the classic stroganoff makes a great winter dinner.

2 tablespoons coconut oil

1 wild rabbit, cut into large pieces

100 g speck, chopped

1 large red onion, chopped

4 garlic cloves, crushed

1 tablespoon smoked paprika

2 teaspoons fennel seeds

800 g can crushed tomatoes

2 cups beef stock (see recipe on page 135)

1 cup red wine

1 red capsicum, thinly sliced

sea salt and ground black pepper

¼ cup chopped flat-leaf parsley

1. Put the coconut oil in a large saucepan over a high heat. When it's hot, brown the rabbit in batches, for 2 minutes each, or until very golden on all sides. Transfer the cooked meat to a heat-proof bowl.

2. Turn the heat down to medium and add the speck and onion. Cook, stirring occasionally, for 3 minutes, or until softened and starting to turn golden. Stir in the garlic, paprika, fennel seeds, tomatoes, stock and wine and bring to a simmer.

3. Return the rabbit and any resting juices to the pan and stir well, then let it simmer, partially covered, for 1 hour. Take off the lid and add the capsicum, then simmer for 10 minutes. Season to taste, then take the pan off the heat and stir the parsley through before serving.

TIP: This is delicious served with our sauerkraut – see the recipe on page 118.

Quail Scotch Eggs

Makes 12

Back in vogue again, scotch eggs are a classic English pub favourite. Packed with flavour, they make a delicious snack or, if you eat enough of them, a tasty meal. This paleo version more than lives up to the original.

600 g fatty pork mince

1 tablespoon wholegrain mustard

1 small red chilli, seeded, finely chopped

2 tablespoons finely chopped chives

1 egg yolk

sea salt and ground black pepper

12 quail eggs

2 cups almond meal

sauerkraut (see recipe on page 118), to serve

1. Line two large baking trays with baking paper, then put the mince, mustard, chilli, chives and egg yolk together in a bowl and mix well. Season, then divide the mixture into 12 and flatten each portion out into a round in the palm of your hand.
2. Put a quail egg on top of the flattened pork mixture in your palm, right in the middle, then carefully fold the meat over to cover the egg. Press the edges tightly together to seal the egg in. Put the almond meal in a bowl, then roll the scotch eggs in it until they're evenly coated. Put the scotch eggs on one of the trays and chill for 1 hour, until firmly set.
3. Preheat the oven to 220°C. Transfer the chilled eggs to the second tray.
4. Bake the scotch eggs for 20–25 minutes, or until the meat is cooked through and golden. Serve warm or at room temperature with sauerkraut.

TIP: It's possible to use chicken eggs instead. Place the eggs in cold water and bring to boil on a high heat. Remove from heat but leave the eggs in the pot with the lid on for 3 minutes. Remove the eggs and submerge them in an ice bath, then continue from step 2.

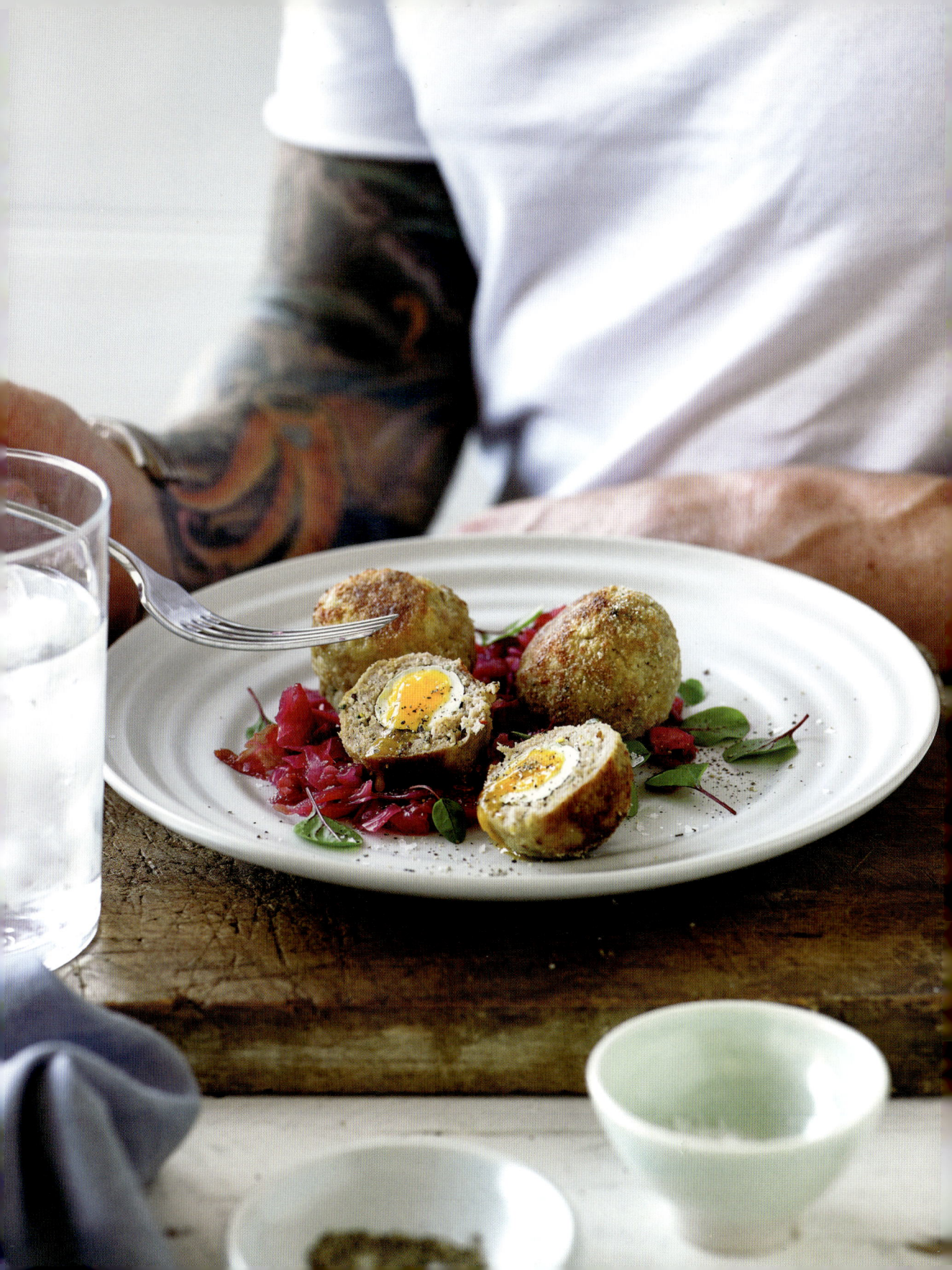

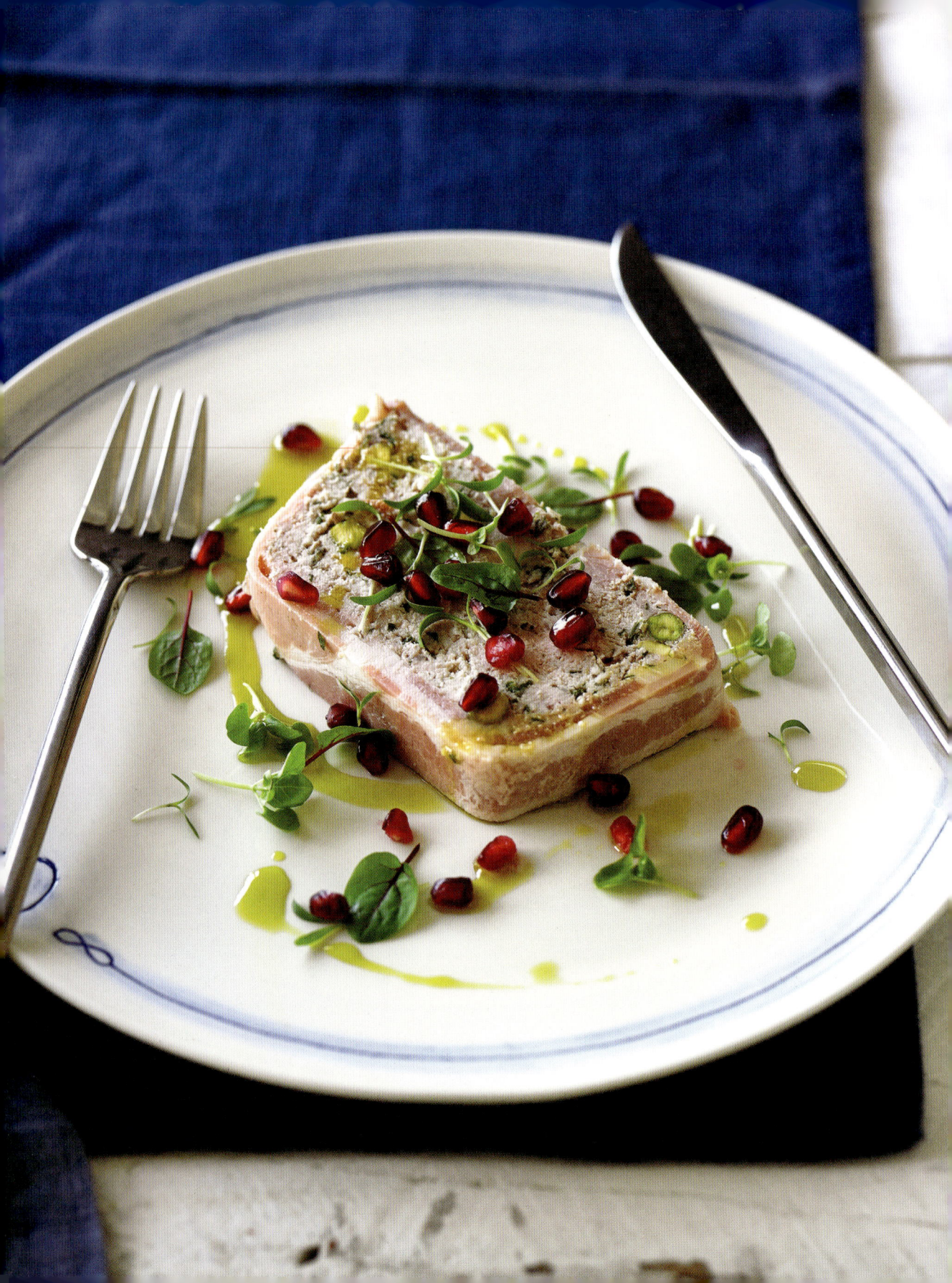

Pork and Pistachio Terrine

Serves 10

Not only does it look impressive when you're having a dinner party, this terrine is high in protein and so easy to make!

8 large rashers rindless bacon

150 g speck, chopped

500 g pork mince

300 g turkey mince

⅔ cup pistachios

2 tablespoons finely chopped sage

¼ cup finely chopped flat-leaf parsley

2 tablespoons thyme leaves

1 tablespoon finely grated lemon zest

¼ cup orange juice

1 egg, lightly whisked

sea salt and ground black pepper

pomegranate seeds, to serve

micro herbs, to serve

avocado oil, to drizzle

1. Preheat your oven to 160°C. Lay the bacon rashers crosswise down the length of a 10 × 20 cm loaf tin, making sure that they overlap slightly and that the ends hang over the edge of the tin.
2. Put all the remaining ingredients together in a bowl, then season to taste and mix until well combined. Press the mixture firmly into the tin and level the surface. Fold the overhanging bacon pieces in to cover the top. Cover the tin with a sheet of baking paper, then with a double sheet of foil to make it airtight.
3. Set the terrine in a deep roasting pan, then half-fill the pan with boiling water. Bake in the oven for 1 hour, then turn the heat down to 140°C and cook for a further 30 minutes, or until the juices run clear when a skewer is inserted in the centre. If the juices are tinged pink, return the terrine to the oven for a further 15 minutes, or until the juices run clear.
4. Take the terrine out of the water bath and put it on a baking tray. Put another baking tray on top, then set 2 heavy cans on top of the tray to weigh it down. Let the terrine cool to room temperature, then put it in the fridge (still with the tray and cans on top) for 6 hours, or overnight if time permits. Serve sliced, with pomegranate seeds and micro herbs and drizzled with avocado oil.

Coconut Berry Tartlets

Makes 4

There's no better combination than berries and coconut – phenomenal! These tartlets are best made with fresh berries, but frozen berries will work too. Just remember to defrost them a little before you serve dessert.

Base

¼ cup sunflower seeds

¼ cup golden linseeds

¼ cup macadamias

¼ cup almond meal

1 tablespoon chia seeds

½ cup pitted dates

½ vanilla bean, seeds scraped

½ teaspoon ground cinnamon

2 tablespoons coconut oil

Filling

250 g whipped coconut cream
   (see recipe on page 130)

1 cup mixed berries

1. To make the base, put all the ingredients together in a food processor and process until smooth. The mix should stick together when pressed, but you don't want it to be too wet or sticky, as it won't hold together. If it isn't sticky enough, add some extra coconut oil. If it's too wet, add more almond meal.

2. Divide the mix between four individual tart tins with loose bases, then press the mixture into the base and up the side of each tin to form a tart shell. Put the tins in the freezer to firm up the bases.

3. To serve, take the tart cases out of the freezer, remove them from the tins, and then gently spoon in the whipped coconut cream and top with the berries. Delicious!

TIP: Instead of using small tartlet tins with loose bases, try making a large version in a pie tin for your next party or celebration.

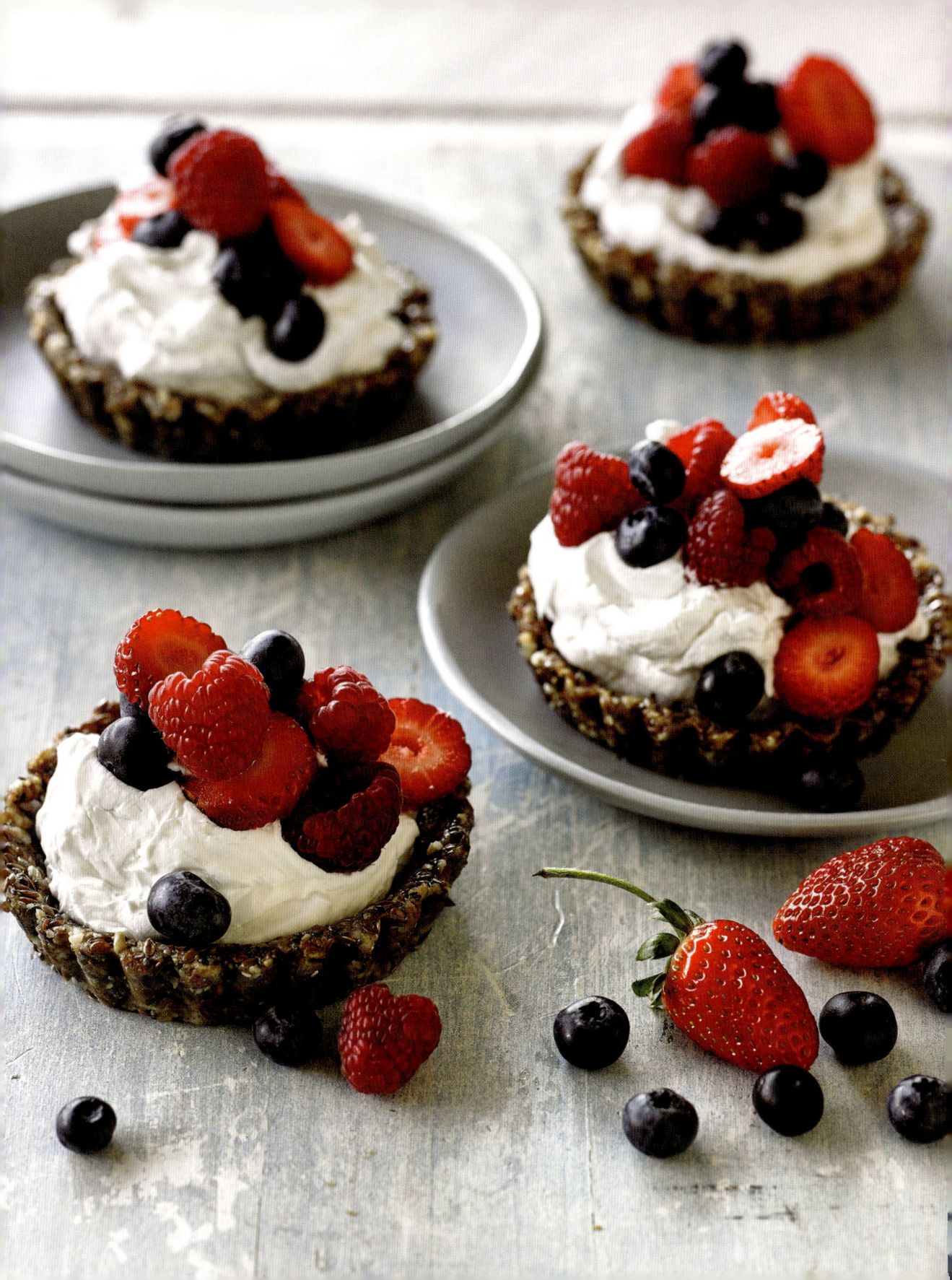

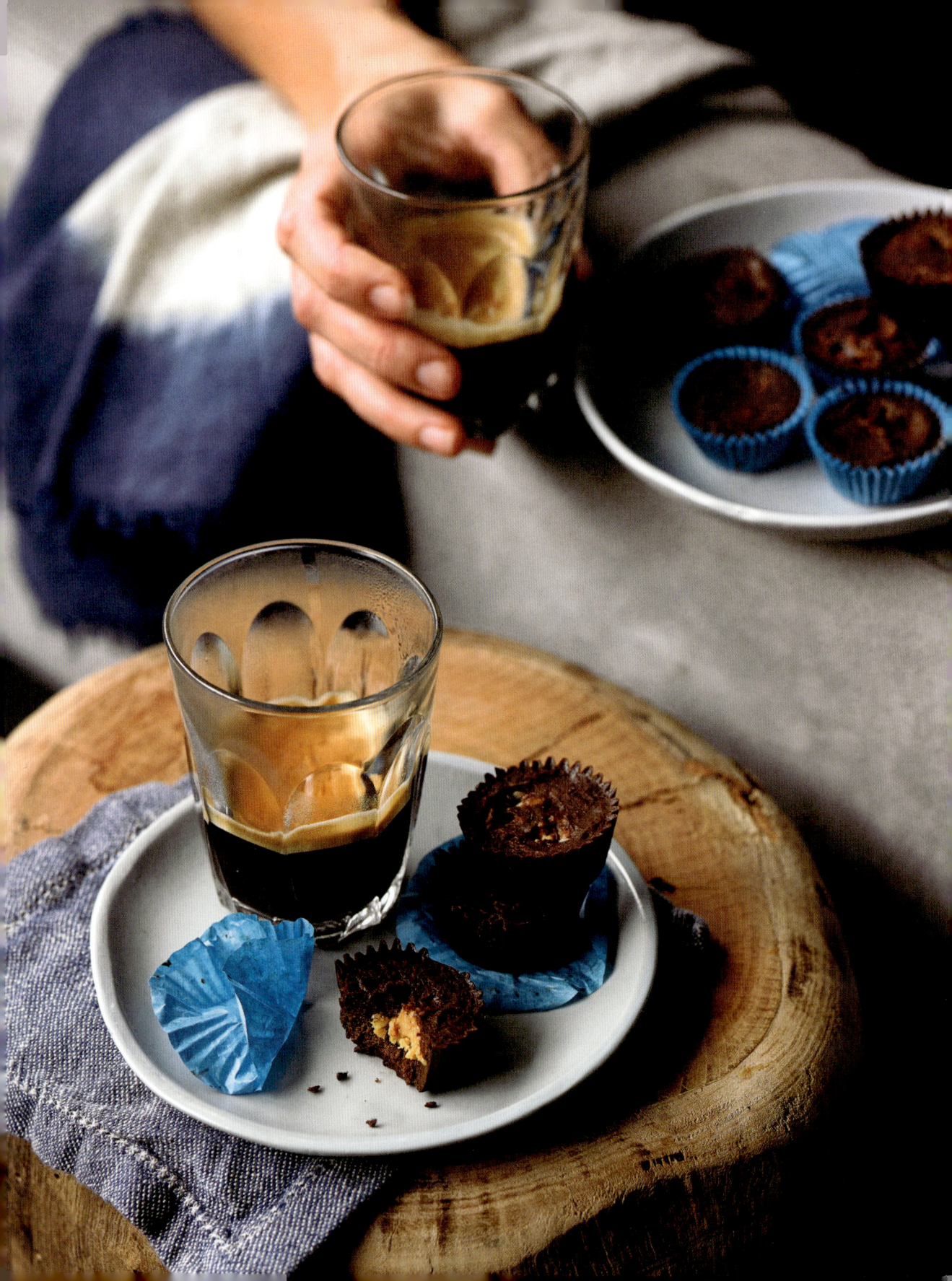

Hazelnut Butter Cups

Makes 12

We're all familiar with Reese's Peanut Butter Cups. Our version, made with hazelnut butter, is a great alternative for next time you're snuggling up on the couch and want a little treat while watching a movie. Quick to make and packed full of nutrients, you can't go wrong with these babies.

½ cup raw cacao powder

¼ cup honey

½ cup coconut oil

2 teaspoons ground cinnamon

pinch of sea salt

½ cup hazelnut butter (raw or roasted)

1. Line a mini cupcake tray with 24 paper or foil patty cases.
2. To make your chocolate, put the cacao, honey, coconut oil, cinnamon and salt in a saucepan over a low heat and stir until smooth.
3. Drop 1 tablespoon of the melted chocolate into each patty case, then smooth the chocolate up the side with the back of your spoon. Put the tray into the freezer for about 10 minutes to set.
4. Take the tray out of the freezer and add 1 teaspoon of the hazelnut butter to each cup. Cover with the remaining melted chocolate, filling each cup almost to the top of the patty case.
5. Set in the fridge or freezer until firm and ready to eat.

Chilled Lemon Curd Creams

Serves 6

When paired with fresh blueberries, these great little lemon curd creams are the perfect dessert to cure those sweet-tooth cravings.

2 eggs, at room temperature

2 egg yolks, at room temperature

¾ cup rice syrup

100 g chilled butter, chopped

juice and finely grated zest of
 2 lemons

400 ml can coconut cream

blueberries, to serve

sliced natural almonds, to serve

1. Whisk the eggs, egg yolks and rice syrup together in a heat-proof bowl until well combined and slightly pale. Transfer the mixture to a saucepan over a medium-low heat and add the butter, lemon juice and zest. Cook, whisking constantly, for 6–8 minutes, or until thick and smooth.

2. Pour the hot lemon mixture back into the same heat-proof bowl, then whisk in the coconut cream. Pour the coconut lemon mixture into six 200 ml serving glasses or jars. Chill in the fridge for 2 hours, or until softly set. Serve topped with blueberries and flaked almonds.

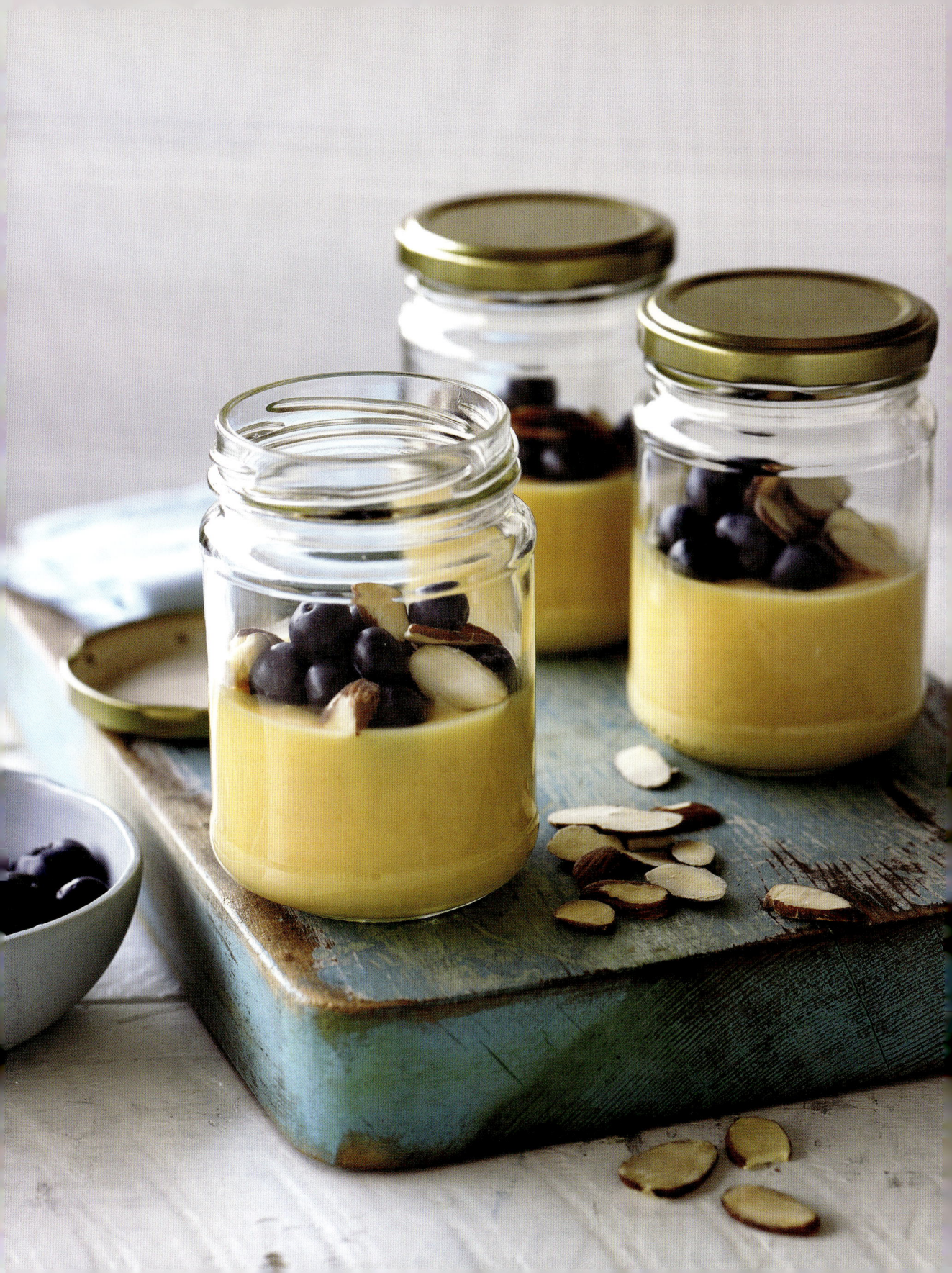

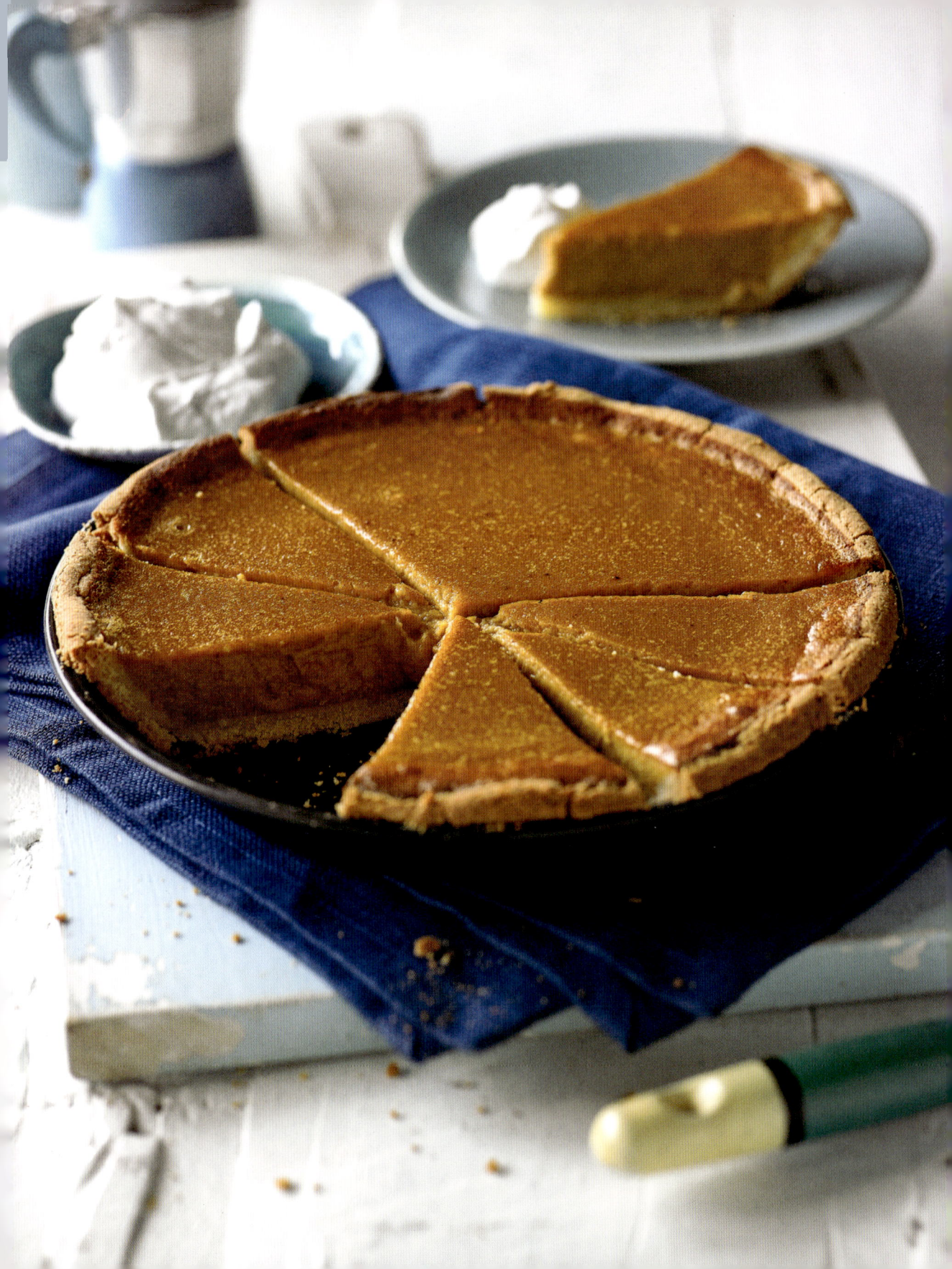

Sweet Pumpkin Pie

Serves 8

This paleo pumpkin pie is full of gorgeous spices that will fill your house with the most delicious scent!

Pumpkin Filling

400 g peeled, seeded butternut pumpkin

2 eggs, at room temperature

2 egg yolks, at room temperature

400 ml can coconut cream

½ cup maple syrup

1½ teaspoons ground cinnamon

½ teaspoon ground ginger

¼ teaspoon ground cloves

Pie Crust

1½ cups almond meal

½ cup coconut flour

½ cup arrowroot

100 g chilled butter, chopped

1 egg, chilled

whipped coconut cream, to serve (see recipe on page 130)

1. To make the pumpkin filling, steam the pumpkin for 8–10 minutes, or until tender. Let it cool, then process until smooth. Add the remaining filling ingredients and process until smooth, then cover the mixture and put it in the fridge.

2. To make the pie crust, grease a 23 cm pie tin, then process the almond meal, coconut flour and arrowroot until combined. Add the butter and process until fine crumbs form. Add the egg and process until the mixture just starts to come together in a ball. Roll the dough out between two sheets of baking paper into a round 4 mm thick. Transfer the pastry to the pie tin and press it firmly into the base and up the side. Trim the edge, then put the tin in the fridge to chill the pie crust for 1 hour or until the pastry is firm.

3. Put a baking tray in the oven and preheat it to 180°C.

4. Take the pie crust out of the fridge and pour in the pumpkin mixture. Level the surface, then put the pie tin in the oven on the preheated tray. Set a timer to go off after 35 minutes.

5. When the timer goes off, cover the pie with a piece of greased foil, then put it back in the oven for a further 35 minutes, or until the pumpkin mixture has set. You can check this by shaking the pie gently – if the centre is wobbly, it's not done yet. Let the pie cool in the tin, then serve it sliced with the whipped coconut cream.

Chargrilled Coconut Waffles

Makes 8

Don't order a stack of heavy waffles from the cafe next door – make these awesome coconut waffles at home instead! They're simple, and they taste great.

½ cup coconut flour

½ cup arrowroot

¼ cup desiccated coconut

2 teaspoons baking powder

1 vanilla bean, seeds scraped

1 cup coconut milk

3 eggs, at room temperature, lightly whisked

1 tablespoon lemon juice

2 tablespoons maple syrup, plus extra to serve

coconut oil, for cooking

sliced banana, to serve

1. Preheat a large chargrill pan over a medium-low heat.

2. Put the coconut flour, arrowroot, coconut, baking powder and vanilla seeds together in a bowl and whisk until well combined. Make a well in the centre and add all the remaining ingredients except the coconut oil and banana. Slowly whisk them together until well combined and smooth, then let the mixture stand for 5 minutes, or until it thickens.

3. Generously grease the preheated chargrill pan with coconut oil, then pour ¼ cup measures of the batter onto the pan to make 9 cm rounds. Cook, in batches, for 1–2 minutes on each side, or until cooked through and golden. Serve the waffles warm with banana and extra maple syrup.

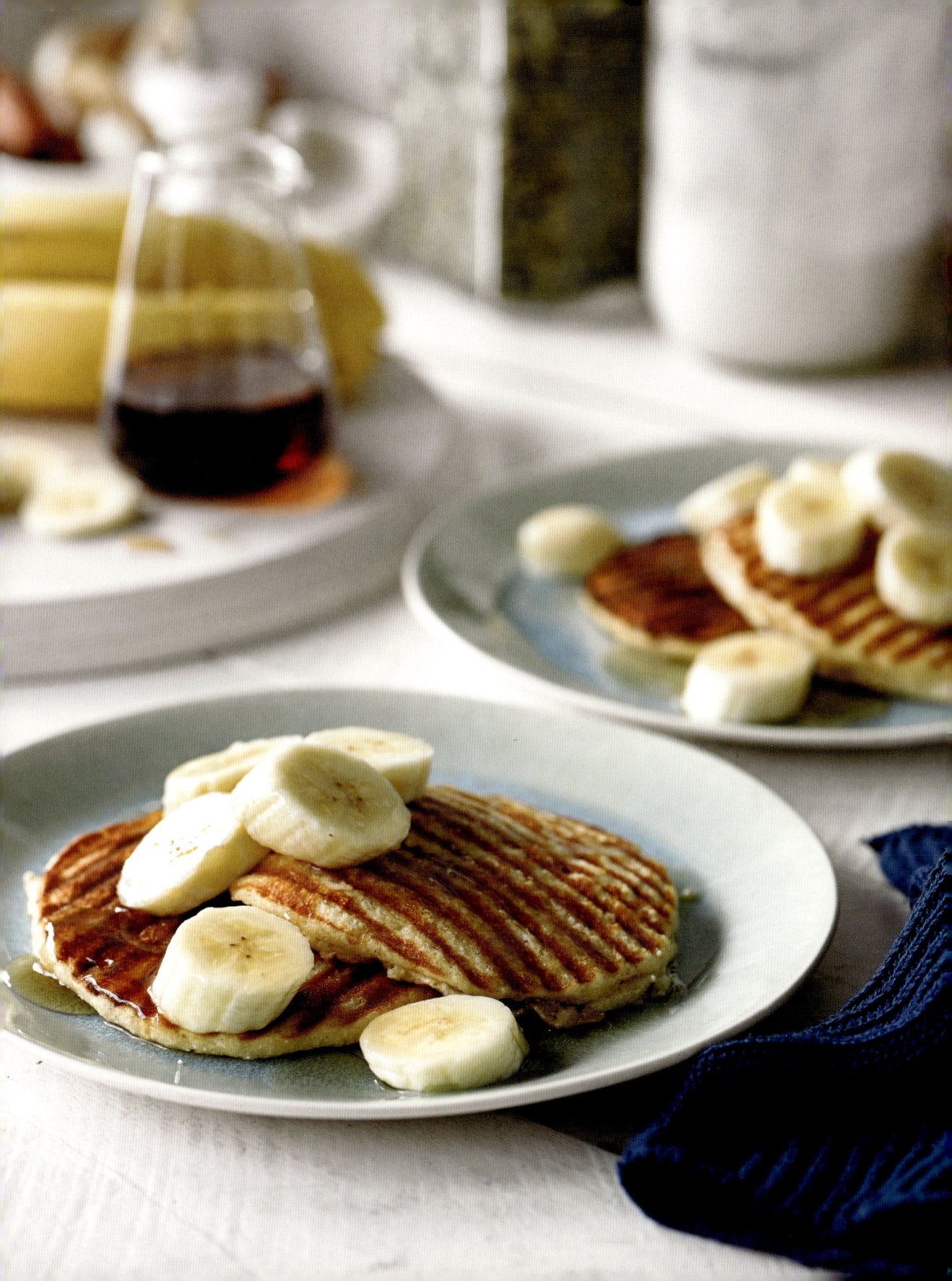

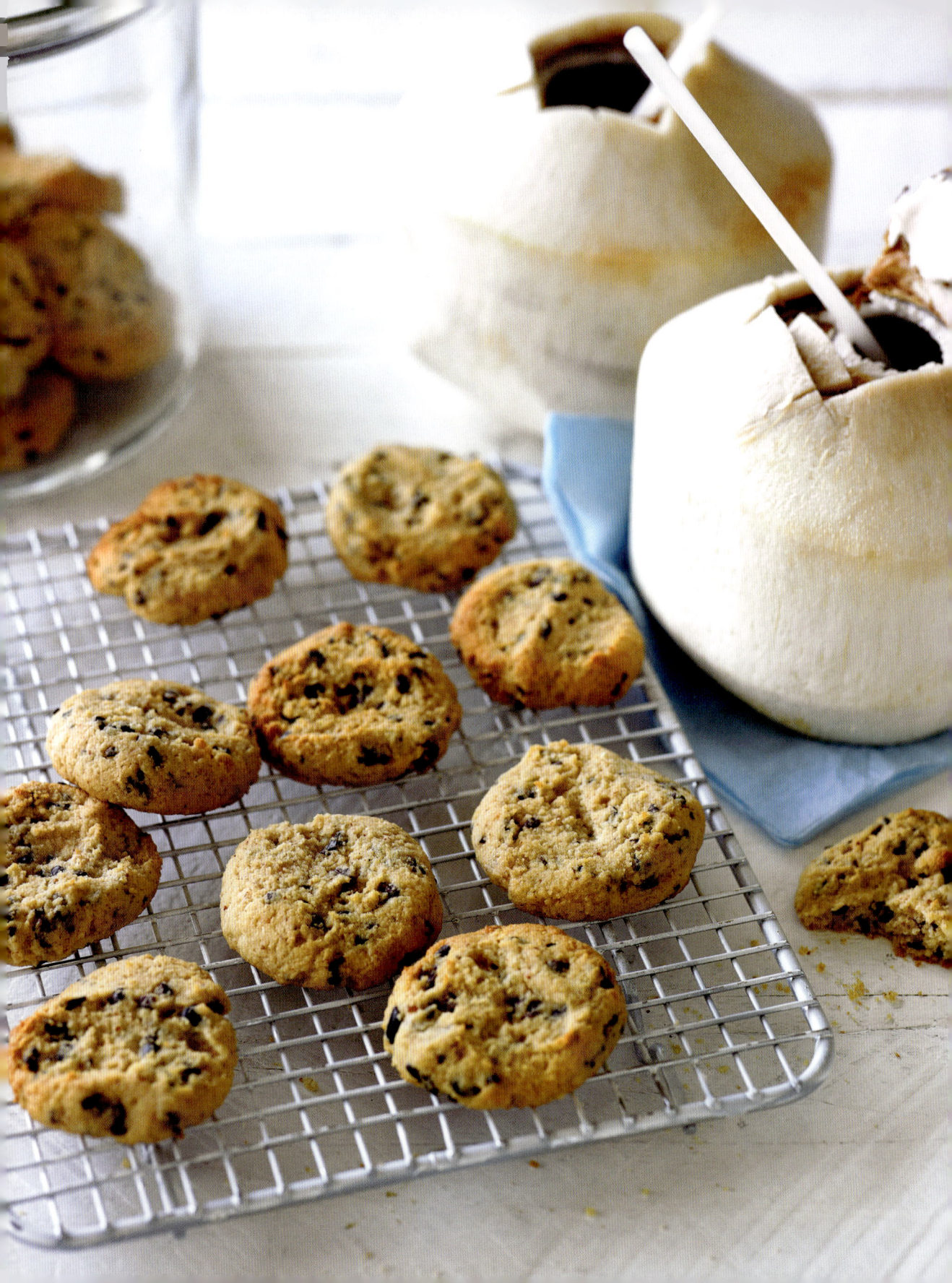

Cacao Chip Cookies

Makes 24

Sometimes you want a simple pick-me-up snack. Put down that packet of store-bought bikkies full of preservatives and other baddies, and instead make a batch of these little cookies. They are just as delicious and much better for you.

100 g butter, at room temperature

⅓ cup almond butter

⅓ cup maple syrup

2 eggs, at room temperature, lightly whisked

½ cup coconut flour

½ cup arrowroot

2 teaspoons baking powder

½ cup raw cacao chips

1. Preheat your oven to 180°C and line two large baking trays with baking paper.
2. Using an electric mixer, whisk the butter, almond butter and maple syrup together in a large bowl until well combined and pale, then add the eggs and whisk again until well combined. Add the coconut flour, arrowroot, baking powder and cacao chips, then stir until well combined.
3. Take 1 tablespoon of the mixture and roll it into a ball, then place it on one of the trays. Repeat with the remaining mixture, placing the balls 4 cm apart. Using your fingertips, push down on the dough balls to flatten them into 5 cm rounds.
4. Bake each tray in the middle of the oven for 10–12 minutes, or until the cookies are cooked through and golden around the edges. Let them stand for 3 minutes on the trays, then transfer to wire racks. Serve warm or at room temperature.

Self-Saucing Cacao Pudding

Serves 4

The great thing about this pudding is that you can easily see the oozy fudgy sauce on top, unlike the traditional version with the sauce at the bottom of the pudding dish. Don't be alarmed at how messy the pudding looks before you put it in the oven – it will look delicious when it's done, we promise!

½ cup coconut flour

2 tablespoons arrowroot

2 tablespoons raw cacao powder, plus 2 tablespoons extra

¼ cup maple syrup, plus ⅓ cup extra

½ cup unsweetened almond milk

2 eggs, at room temperature, lightly whisked

50 g butter, melted and cooled

whipped coconut cream, to serve (see recipe on page 130)

1. Preheat your oven to 180°C. Grease a 4-cup capacity round heat-proof dish.
2. Put the coconut flour, arrowroot and cacao together in a bowl and whisk until well combined. Make a well in the centre and add the maple syrup, almond milk, eggs and butter, then slowly whisk together until well combined and smooth. Spoon the mixture into the dish and level the surface.
3. Sprinkle the extra cacao evenly over the surface of the batter, then drizzle evenly with the extra maple syrup. Pour 200 ml of boiling water carefully over the back of a large metal spoon onto the surface, covering the cacao and maple syrup mixture evenly.
4. Put the pudding in the oven to bake for 30 minutes, or until the sauce on top is thick and fudgy. Serve immediately with the whipped coconut cream.

TIP: Make sure everyone is ready and waiting for this pudding, as it's best served straight from the oven. If left to stand, the cakey part of the pudding will slowly soak up the delicious fudgy sauce on top.

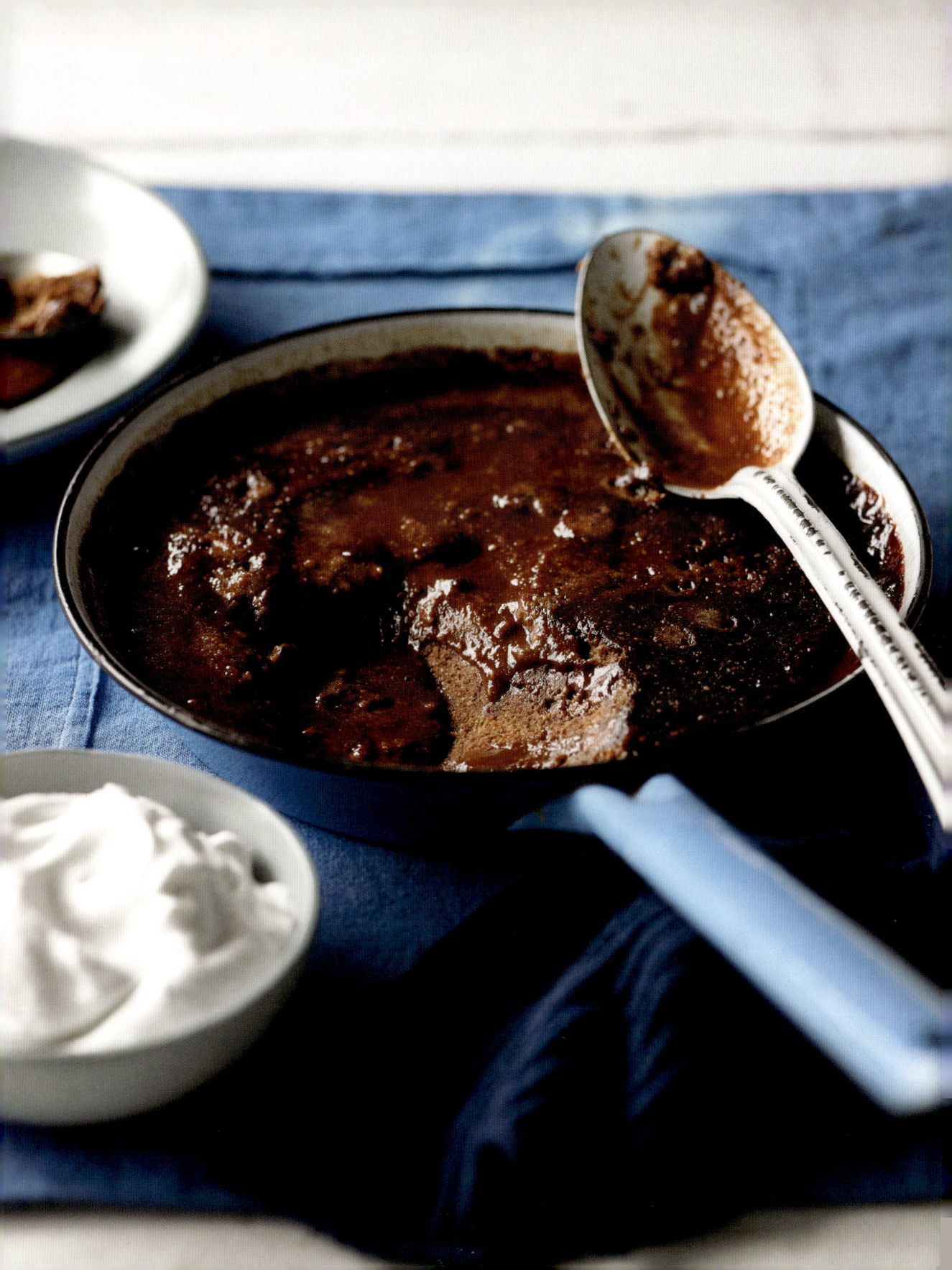

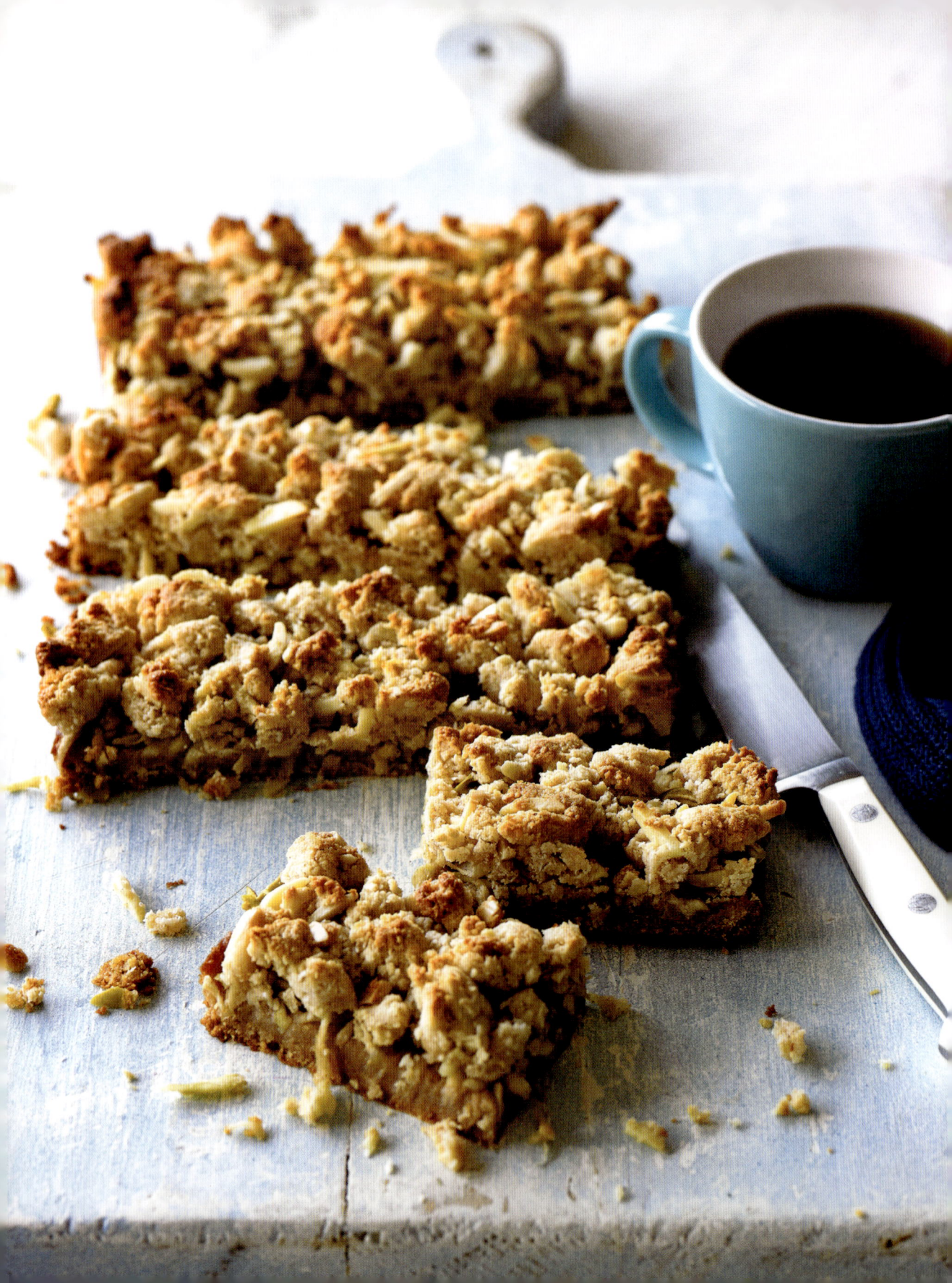

Apple Crumble Slice

Serves 8

Aussies love a crumble in winter, and there's no reason to go without just because you're eating clean. With this trusty recipe you can skip all that added sugar!

2½ cups almond meal

¼ cup arrowroot

⅓ cup maple syrup

1 teaspoon ground cinnamon

½ teaspoon freshly grated nutmeg

150 g chilled butter, chopped

1 large green apple, cored, coarsely grated

½ cup slivered almonds

½ cup desiccated coconut

1. Preheat your oven to 180°C, then grease a 26 × 16 cm cake tin and line the base and sides with baking paper.

2. Put the almond meal, arrowroot, maple syrup, cinnamon, nutmeg and butter together in a food processor and process until well combined. The mixture will be sticky. Press three-quarters of the mixture into the base of the cake tin and put the remaining mixture in a bowl.

3. Bake the almond meal base for 20 minutes, or until it is cooked around the edges and light golden. Take it out of the oven and top evenly with the apple.

4. Add the slivered almonds and coconut to the remaining almond meal mixture in the bowl. Using your fingertips, rub the mixture together to form large crumbs. Sprinkle the crumb mixture evenly over the apple in the tin, then put it in the oven to bake for 15 minutes, or until cooked and golden brown.

5. Take the tin out of the oven and let it cool to room temperature, then chill in the fridge for 1 hour, or until firm, before serving.

Raspberry Coconut Truffles

Makes 28

A fantastic alternative to that mid-afternoon chocolate bar, these little truffles taste great and are incredibly more-ish.

1 tablespoon chia seeds

1½ cups raw cashews

½ cup desiccated coconut

125 g raspberries

2 tablespoons rice syrup

1 tablespoon coconut oil

2 vanilla beans, seeds scraped

raw cacao powder

1. Line a large baking tray with baking paper.
2. Whisk the chia seeds with 2 tablespoons of water and set them aside for 20 minutes, or until plump and translucent.
3. Meanwhile, cover the cashews with boiling water. Let them stand for 20 minutes to soften, then drain them.
4. Put the chia mixture and cashews in a food processor with the coconut, raspberries, rice syrup, coconut oil and vanilla seeds, then process until well combined and smooth. The mixture will be soft and sticky.
5. Drop level tablespoon measures of the mixture into small mounds on the tray. Chill for 1 hour, or until firm, then roll each mound into a smooth ball. Put the tray back in the fridge and let the truffles chill for 6 hours, or overnight if time permits, until very firm.
6. Lightly roll the truffles in the cacao powder before serving.

TIP: Always keep the truffles chilled so that they remain firm.

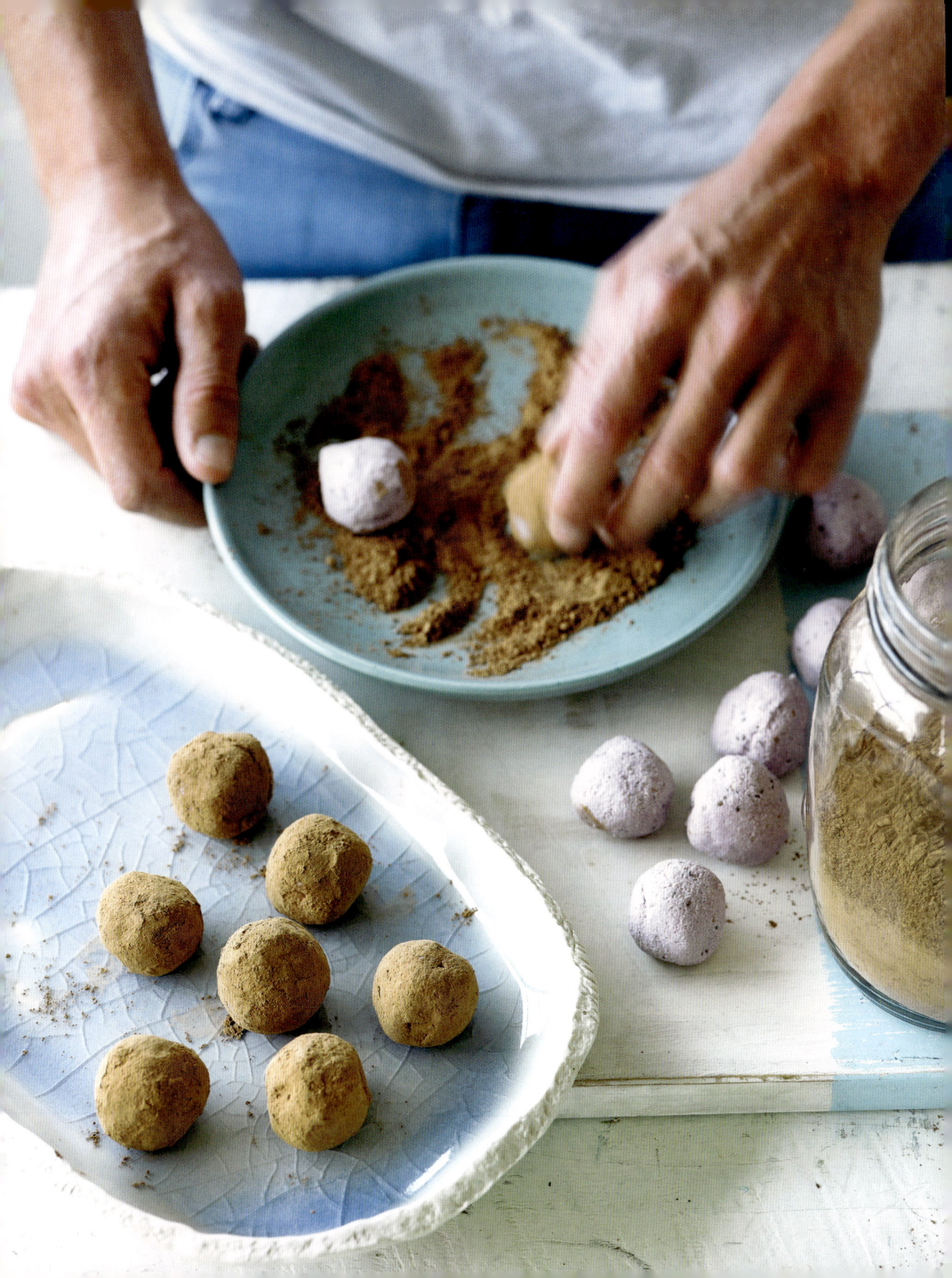

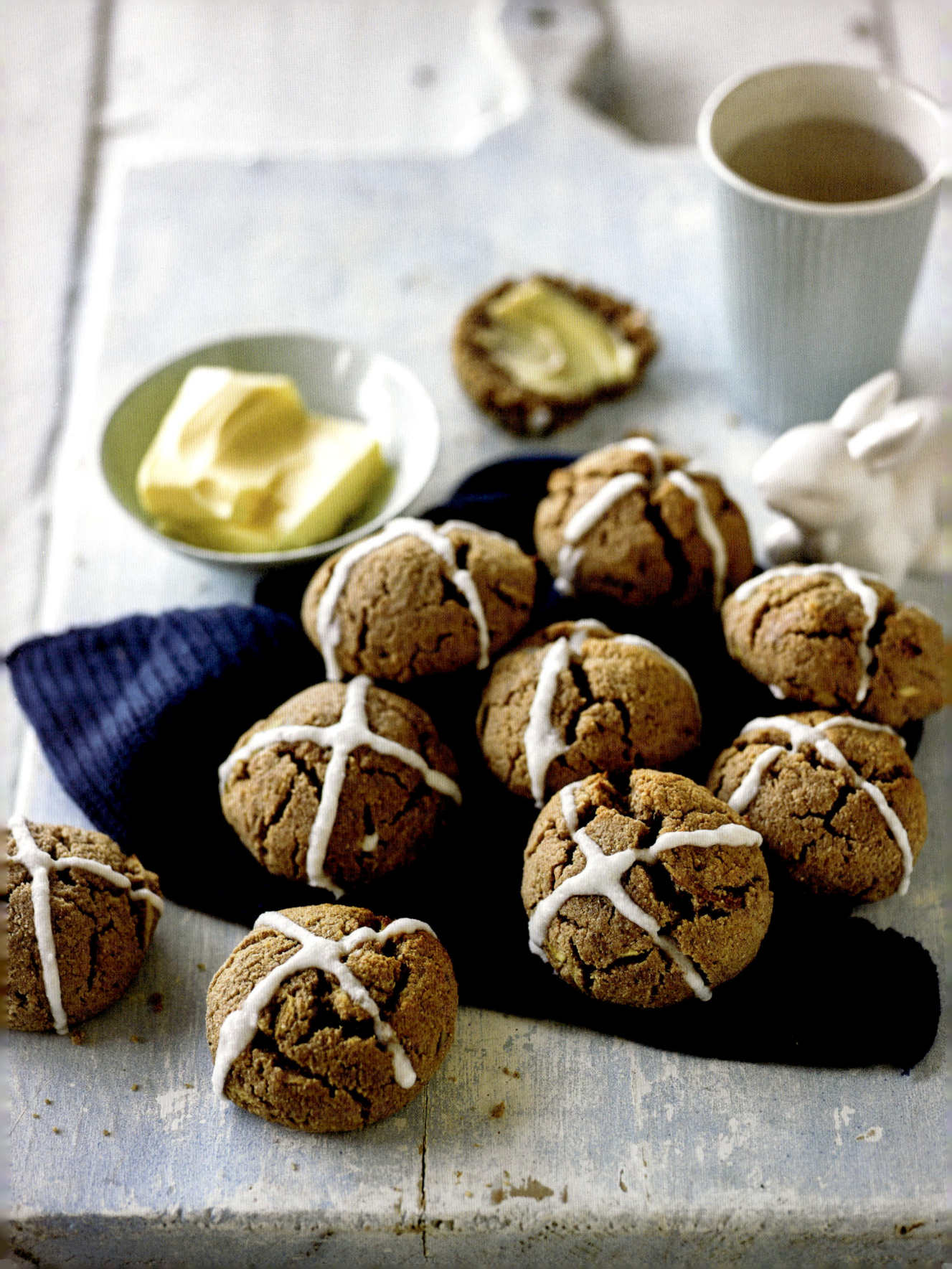

Hot Cross Buns

Makes 12

Instead of stopping by your local bakery, why not knock up a batch of these Easter treats at home? Your body will thank you for choosing the healthy option.

Buns

1 cup almond meal

½ cup coconut flour

½ cup arrowroot

½ cup coarsely grated green apple

2 teaspoons baking powder

3 teaspoons ground cinnamon

2 teaspoons freshly grated nutmeg

½ teaspoon ground cloves

4 eggs, at room temperature, lightly whisked

¼ cup rice syrup

150 g butter, melted and cooled, plus extra to serve

Crosses

2 tablespoons coconut cream

1 tablespoon coconut oil, melted

2 teaspoons coconut flour

1. Preheat your oven to 180°C and line a large baking tray with baking paper.

2. To make the buns, put all the ingredients together in a large bowl and mix well to combine. Stand for 10 minutes or until the mixture is firm. Shape the mixture into 12 rounds and put them on the tray 2 cm apart.

3. Bake the buns for 20 minutes, or until golden. When they're cooked, a skewer inserted in the centre should come out clean. Let the buns cool on the tray for 5 minutes.

4. To make the crosses, put all the ingredients together in a bowl and whisk until smooth, then spoon the mixture into a small zip-lock bag. Snip off one small corner of the bag, then pipe crosses on top of the buns. Chill until set.

5. Serve warm, with extra butter.

Easter Eggs

Makes 16–24

When supermarkets are stacked with Easter eggs, they can be hard to resist. These great little sweets are a much better option, full of creamy caramel but without all that unnecessary sugar and dairy.

Chocolate

¾ cup coconut oil, melted and cooled but runny

⅓ cup raw cacao powder

¼ cup maple syrup

Caramel

½ cup pitted dates, chopped

¼ cup coconut cream

1. To make the chocolate, put the coconut oil, cacao and maple syrup together in a bowl and mix until well combined and smooth. Spoon 1–2 teaspoons of the mixture into each hole of a 16-hole Easter egg mould, then use the back of the spoon to spread it evenly over the base and side of each hole. Set the remaining chocolate aside, then put the mould in the fridge for 15 minutes, or until the eggs are firm.

2. Meanwhile, to make the caramel, put the dates and coconut cream together in a blender and blend until very smooth.

3. Once the chocolate has set in the mould, fill each egg with the caramel mixture and spoon the remaining chocolate mixture over the top of the caramel filling as a seal. Put the filled eggs in the fridge for 1 hour, or until firm. Carefully pop out the Easter eggs and serve chilled.

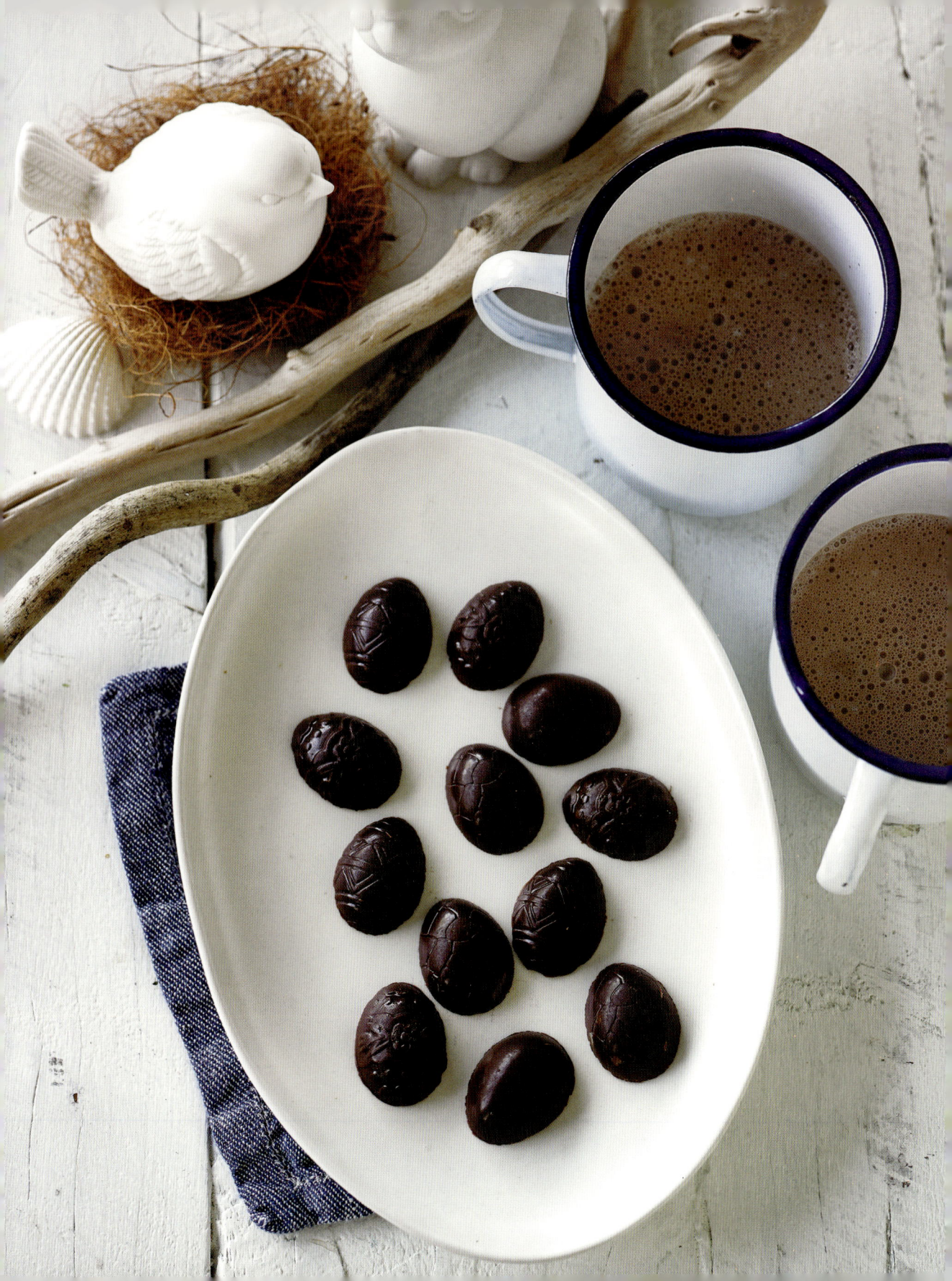

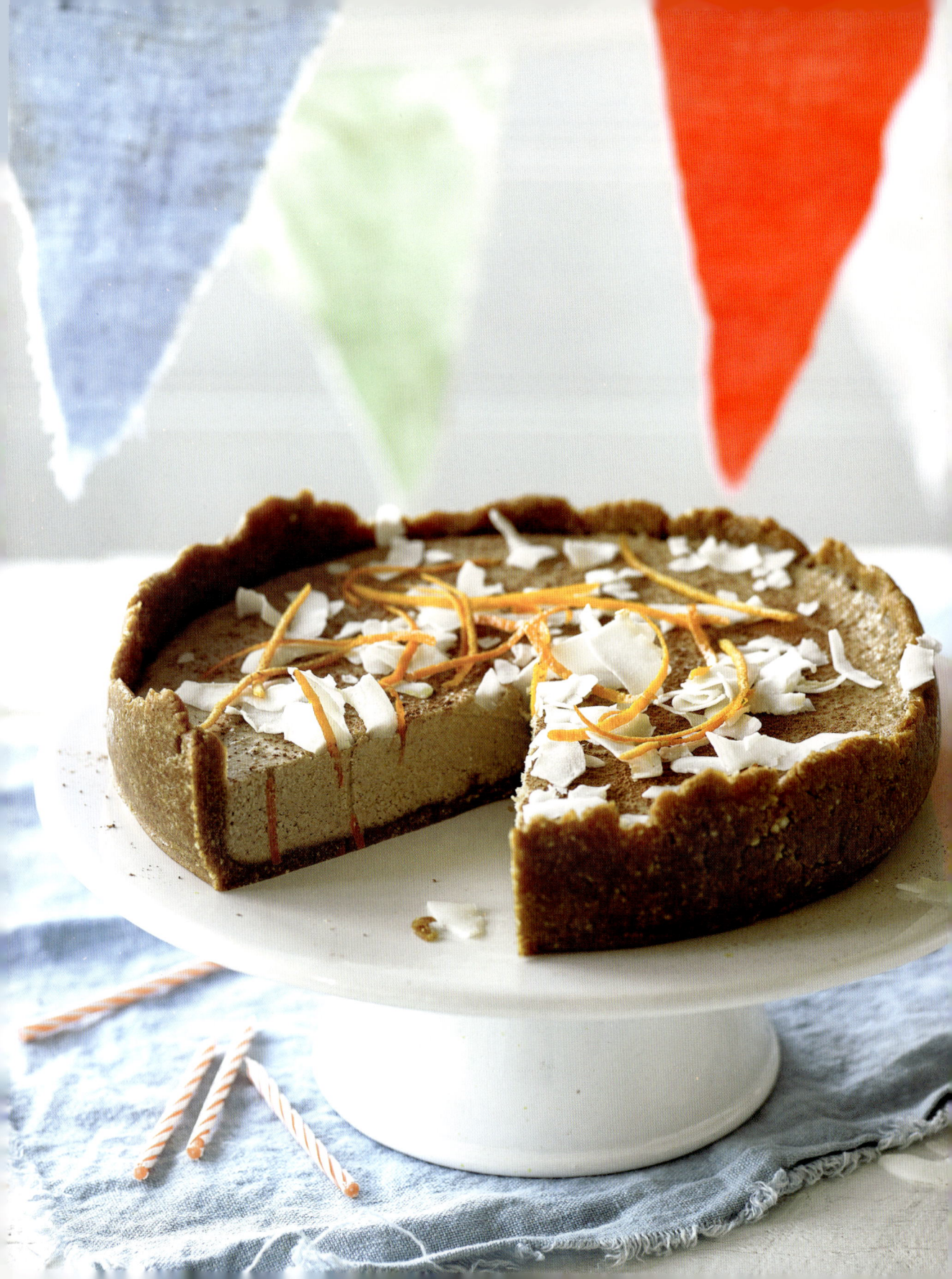

Tess's Spiced Dream Cake

Makes 1 cake

This little gem comes from the amazing Tess from WellnessByTess in Bondi.

Base

180 g pitted dates

1 cup raw almonds

1 cup shredded coconut

¼ cup mesquite powder

pinch of sea salt

1 tablespoon grated ginger

1 teaspoon ground cloves

2 tablespoons orange zest

Filling

2 cups cashews, soaked overnight

½ cup brewed chai tea

½ cup coconut milk

¼ cup maple syrup

⅓ cup cacao butter, melted

⅓ cup coconut oil, melted

¼ cup mesquite powder

2 teaspoons ground cinnamon

½ teaspoon ground cardamom

1 vanilla bean, seeds scraped

3–4 drops orange oil

1. Line a 22 cm springform cake tin with baking paper.

2. To make the base, put all the ingredients in a food processor and process until you have a nice dough. Transfer the dough to the cake tin, then press it firmly into the base and halfway up the side of the tin to form a crust. Let it rest in the fridge while you make the filling.

3. To make the filling, blend all the ingredients together in a food processor, then pour the mixture over the base and put the cake in the freezer to set.

4. Take the cake out of the freezer and leave it in the fridge to soften before it's served. If you like, you can garnish with orange zest strips, coconut flakes and cacao powder.

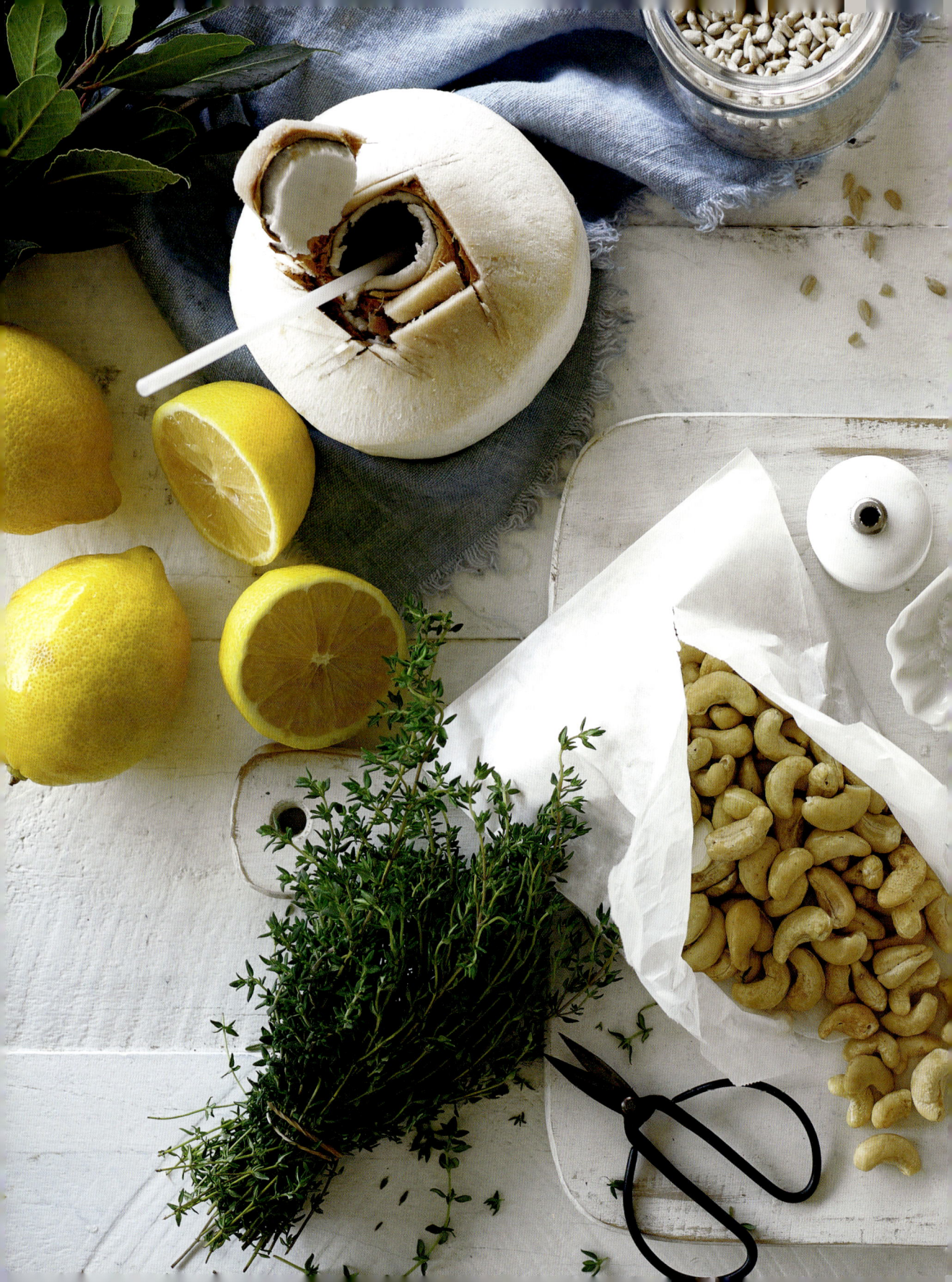

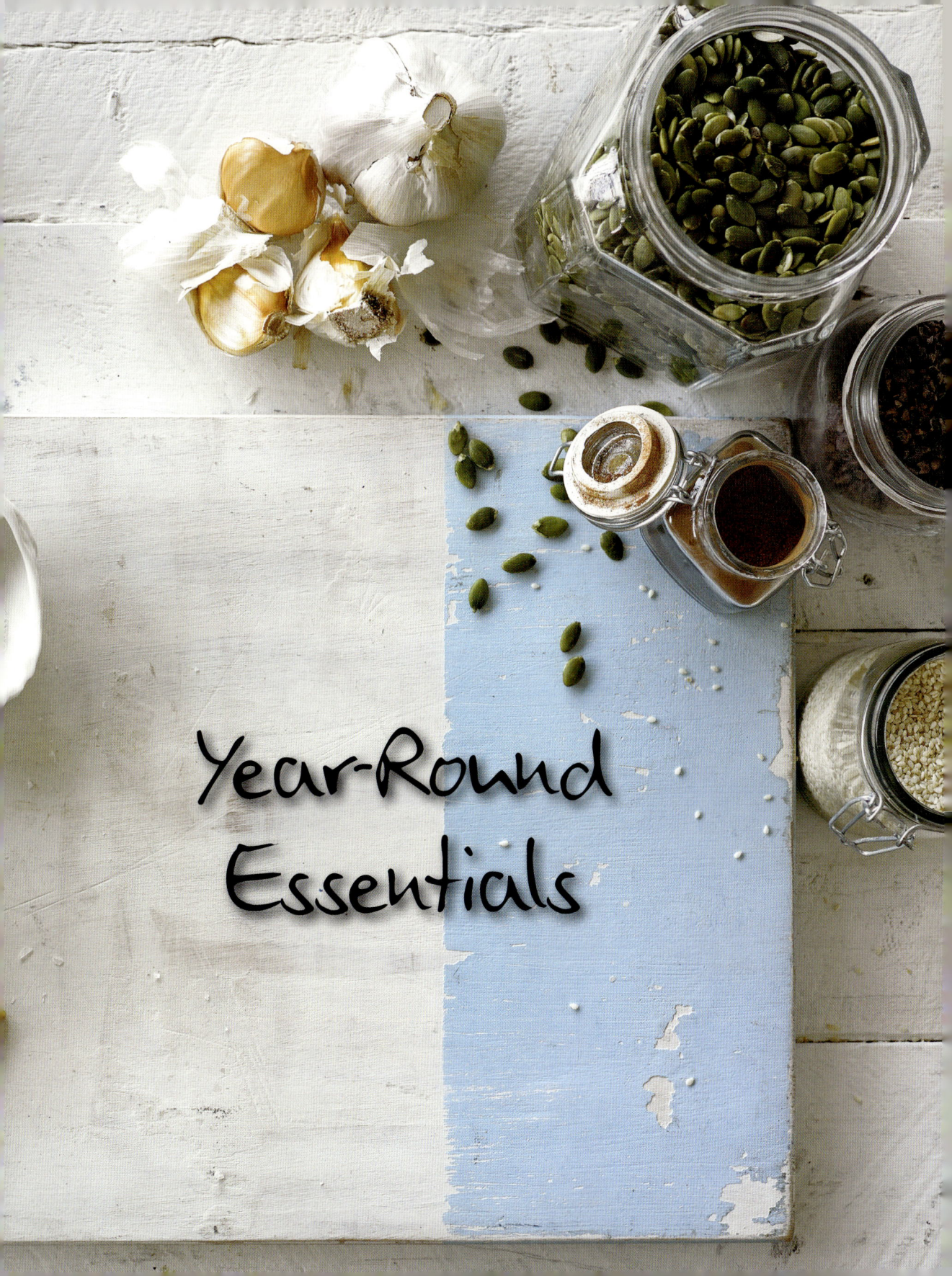

Year-Round
Essentials

Fermented Veggies   117

Sauerkraut   118

Scott's Breakfast   121

Activated Nuts and Seeds   122

Linseed Crackers   125

Port, Peppercorn and Chicken Liver Pâté   126

Luke's Spicy Kale Chips   128

Raw Cashew Sour Cream   129

Garlic Aioli   129

Whipped Coconut Cream   130

Coconut Kefir   131

Minty Tonic for Digestion   132

Easy Chicken Broth   133

Morning Bone Broth   134
Roasted Beef Bone Broth   135
Morning Elixir   136
Beet Kvass   137
Burnt Butter Fat-Washed Iced Coffee   139
Nut Berry Smoothie   140
Green and Orange Smoothie   140
The Go-To Smoothie   141
Green Paws Smoothie   141
Beetroot and Ginger Smoothie   142
Coconut and Kale Kickstart Smoothie   143

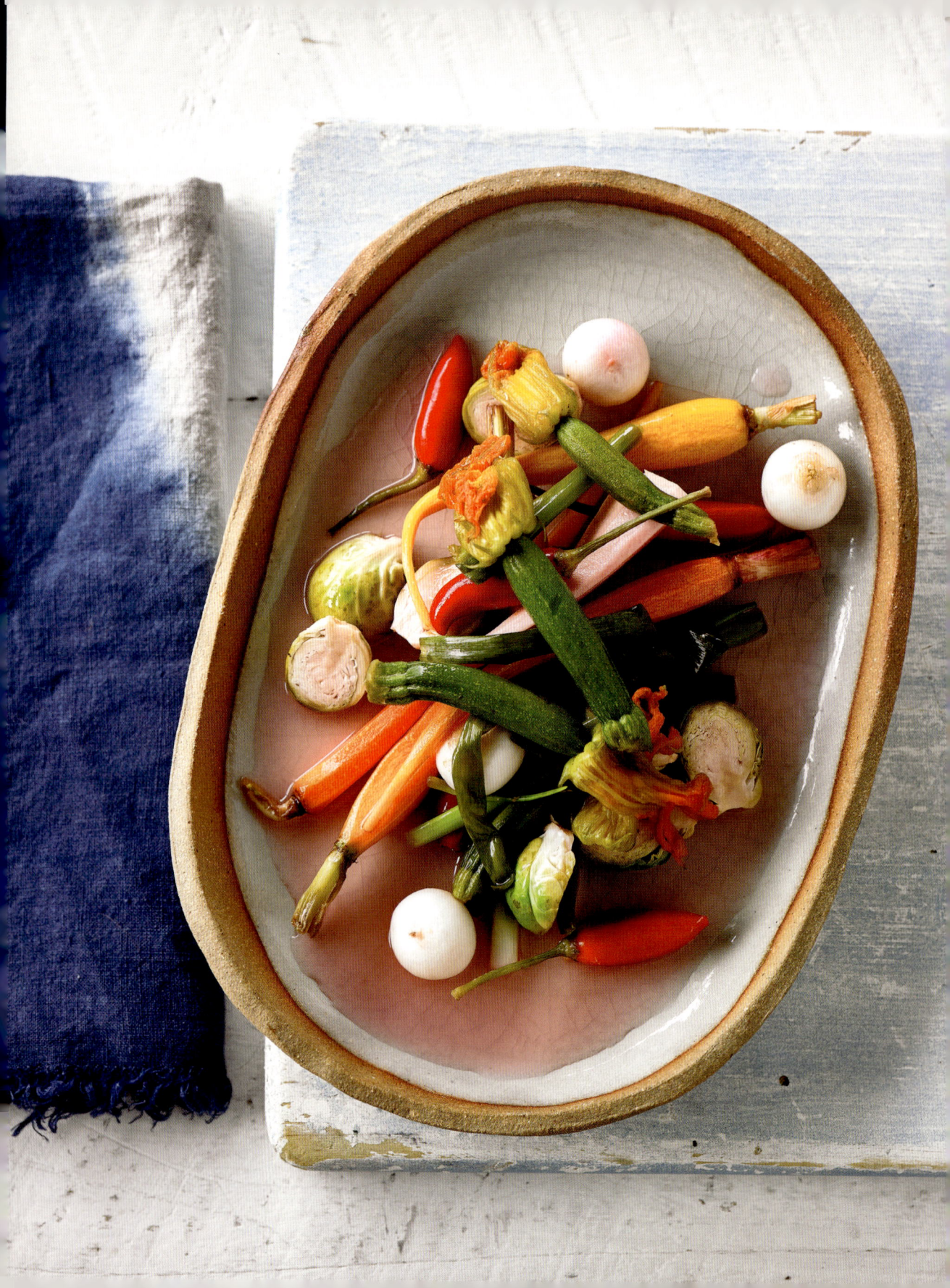

Fermented Veggies

Makes about 4 cups

Fermented veggies are all the rage at the moment, and with good reason – they are full of the probiotics so important for your gut health. We love them as a side for any main meal, but they're great on their own for a quick snack as well.

2 baby parsnips, peeled and quartered lengthwise

250 g baby rainbow carrots, peeled

100 g baby white turnips

150 g baby brussels sprouts, halved lengthwise

8 baby zucchini flowers

6 spring onions, cut into 5 cm lengths

8 small red chillis

¼ cup sea salt

filtered water

1. Put the parsnips, carrots, turnips, brussels sprouts, zucchini flowers, spring onions and chillis in a bowl and toss to combine. Put a small amount of the veggie mixture in a 2 litre sterilised glass jar with an airtight lid.

2. Sprinkle some of the sea salt over the veggies in the jar, then add another layer of veggies and salt, pressing down firmly as you go. Keep going until the jar is nearly full, leaving 5 cm between the top of the veggies and the rim of the jar. Finish with a layer of salt.

3. Pour over enough filtered water to cover the veggies. Put a shot glass on top of the veggies to weigh them down and make sure they are completely covered by the water.

4. Cover the mouth of the jar with a piece of muslin and secure it firmly with a large elastic band. Set the jar aside in a warm spot in your kitchen (the top of the fridge is quite good) and let the veggies ferment for 3–5 days. Check it every day to make sure that the veggies are still covered by the liquid and top it up with more water if necessary.

5. You will know when the veggies are ready by tasting them. When they are done, they'll have a sweet, fermented taste. Discard the muslin cover and put the airtight lid on the jar. Chill until ready to use.

Sauerkraut

Makes about 6 cups

Sauerkraut is a classic fermented side dish and adds an excellent splash of colour to your plate. Serve it with any main meal and your gut bacteria will thank you.

400 g green cabbage, shredded

400 g red cabbage, shredded

2 tablespoons sea salt

filtered water

1. Put a small amount of green and red cabbage into a sterilised 1.5 litre glass jar with an airtight lid.

2. Sprinkle some of the sea salt over the cabbage in the jar and pound it down using the back of a wooden spoon to break down the cabbage and extract some liquid. Add another layer of cabbage and salt, pressing down firmly and pounding as you go. Keep going until the jar is nearly full, leaving 5 cm between the top of the cabbage and the rim of the jar. Finish with a layer of salt.

3. Pour over enough filtered water to cover the cabbage mixture. Put a shot glass on top of the cabbage to weigh it down and make sure it is completely covered by the water.

4. Cover the mouth of the jar with a piece of muslin and secure it firmly with a large elastic band. Set the jar aside in a warm spot in your kitchen (the top of the fridge is quite good) and let the cabbage ferment for 7–10 days. Check it every day to make sure that the cabbage is still covered by the liquid and top it up with more water if necessary.

5. You will know when the cabbage is ready by tasting it. When it is done, it will have a sweet, fermented taste. Discard the muslin cover and put the airtight lid on the jar. Chill until ready to use.

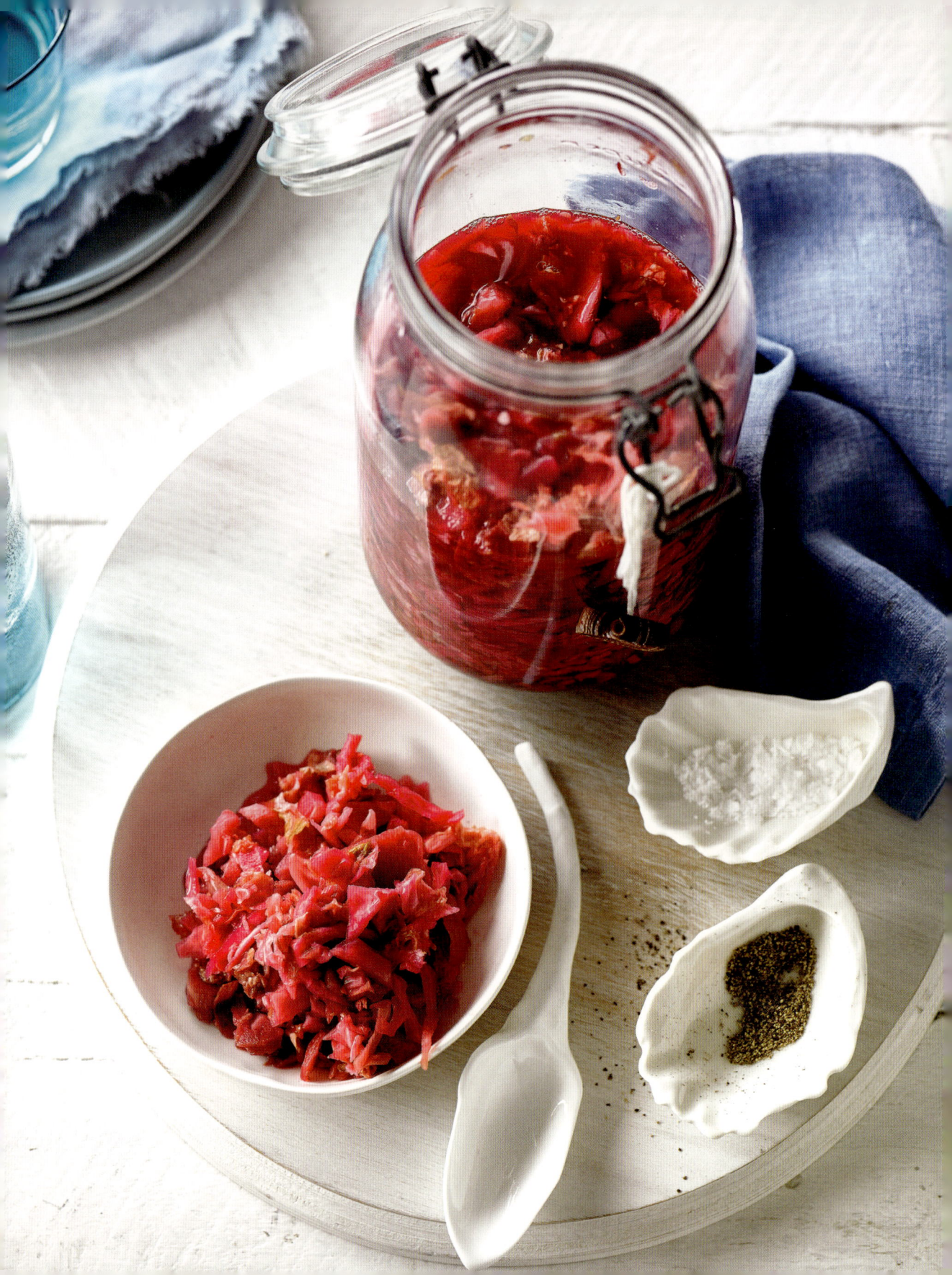

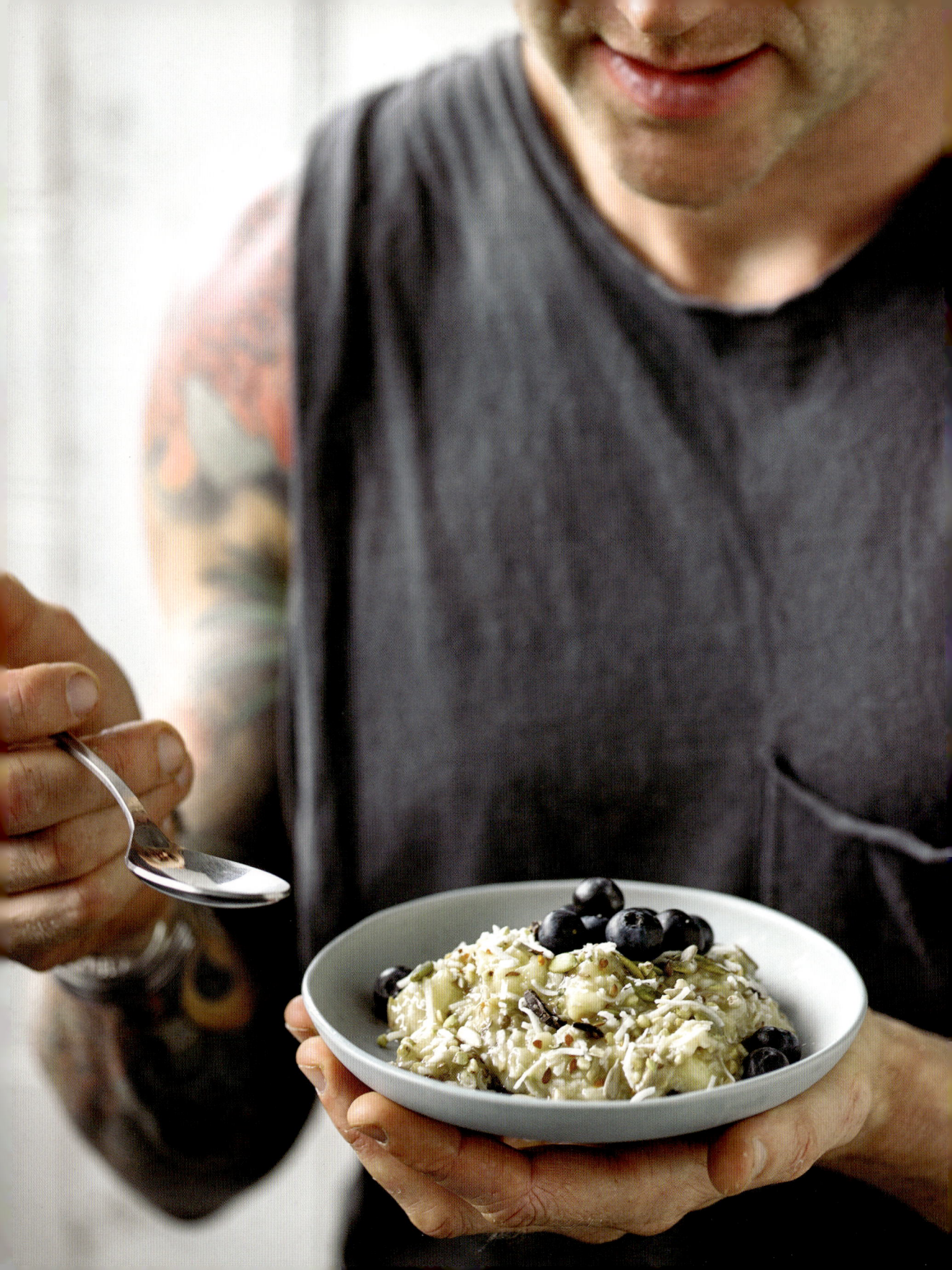

Scott's Breakfast

Makes 1 big batch

Scott says: 'This is the reason I get out of bed in the morning. As a personal trainer, I need a combination of slow-release energy and instant energy to get me through my morning – some instant energy from the banana and berries and some slow-release fuel from the seeds and coconut oil. Make a big batch up in advance to save time and money.'

4 cups shredded coconut

½ cup bee pollen

½ cup pepitas

½ cup linseeds

½ cup sunflower seeds

2 cups hemp seeds

2 cups buckinis

¼ cup cacao nibs

Toppings

1 small banana

1 tablespoon hulled tahini

2 tablespoons coconut oil

blueberries, to serve

1. Mix the coconut, bee pollen, seeds, buckinis and cacao nibs in a large airtight container. Add or omit any ingredients you like and feel free to change the quantities to suit your taste.
2. Mash the banana with the tahini, then add 3–4 tablespoons of the seed mix. Add the coconut oil and then gently mix together to ensure the oil coats the mix. Top with some blueberries.

Activated Nuts and Seeds

Serves 2

There's no reason party nibbles can't be healthy. Nuts and seeds are a delicious and nutritious addition to the paleo way of life. These guys also make a great snack for when you are on the road or away from the kitchen.

500 g raw nuts and/or seeds

filtered water

TIP: Try adding activated nuts to your smoothies or salads for an extra hit of good fats, or grind them into a flour for use in baking.

1. Put the nuts and/or seeds in a bowl. Add enough filtered water to cover them completely, then set aside to soak. Almonds, hazelnuts and brazil nuts need to soak for 12 hours; macadamia nuts, 7–12 hours; pepitas, 7–10 hours; walnuts, 4–8 hours; pecans and pistachios, 4–6 hours; cashews, 2–4 hours; and sunflower seeds, 2 hours.

2. After soaking, the nuts and/or seeds will look swollen and puffy. Drain them and then rinse them under cold running water.

3. Now that you've activated the nutrients in the nuts and/or seeds, you'll need to treat them gently. Toast them in a dehydrator, if you have one, or put them in the oven at the lowest temperature possible (around 50°C). This step will take anywhere from 6 to 24 hours. The nuts and/or seeds are ready when they feel and taste completely dry.

4. After cooling, store the nuts and/or seeds in an airtight container at room temperature.

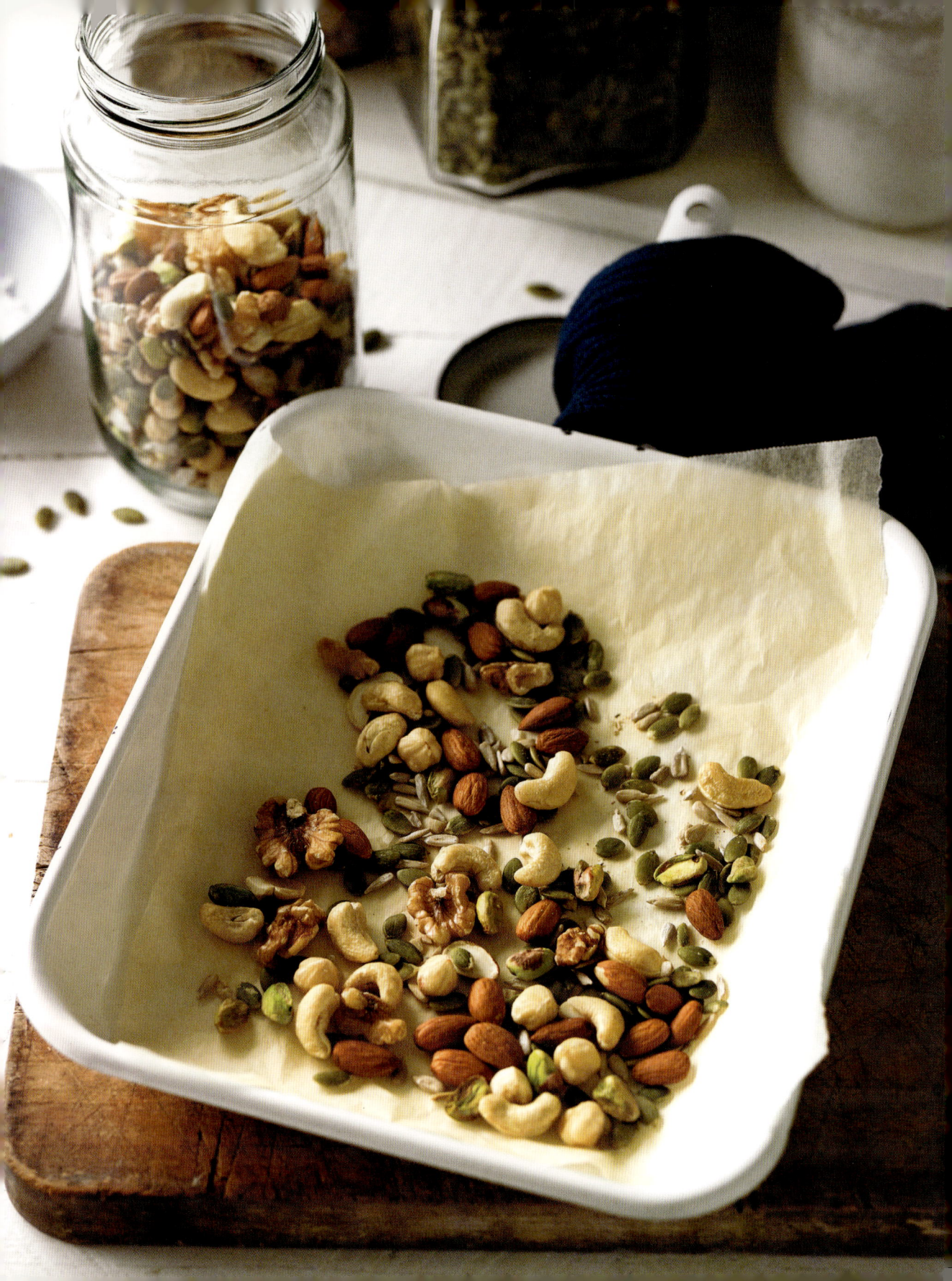

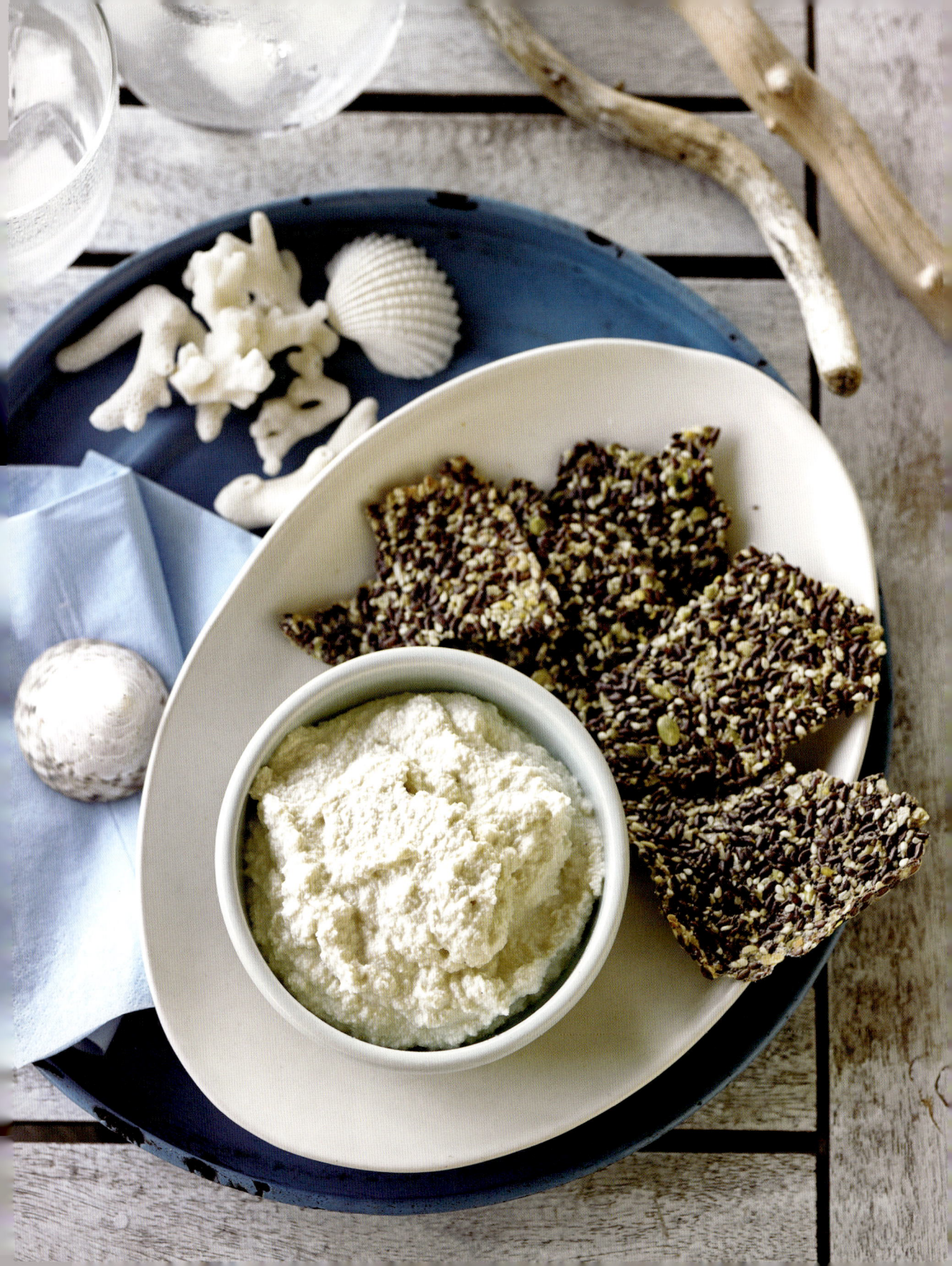

Linseed Crackers

Serves 6

These linseed crackers are a fantastic party nibble or anytime snack. Nutritious and delicious, they are crunchy and nutrient-dense. These crackers are perfect with any kind of dip or pâté. You can even crush them into small pieces and sprinkle them over a salad or poached or scrambled eggs, or use them for nachos.

150 g linseeds

100 g mixed seeds, such as pepitas, sunflower and sesame

½ teaspoon sea salt

1 teaspoon spice, such as cayenne pepper, smoked paprika, ground cumin

TIP: Mix up the flavours and tantalise your tastebuds by playing around with all sorts of different spices! We like making Mexican-inspired crackers and eating them with guacamole.

1. Put the linseeds in a bowl, then pour in enough water to cover them and set them aside. Put the mixed seeds in a separate bowl, pour in enough water to cover them, and then leave both bowls overnight.

2. The next morning, drain the linseeds, which will have a jelly-like texture, then drain and rinse the mixed seeds. Add the mixed seeds to the linseeds, then add the salt and spice and transfer the mixture to a blender. Pulse a few times to break up the seeds, but don't overdo it. You want the seeds to be ground up but still a little chunky.

3. Preheat your oven to 50°C and line two baking trays with baking paper. Spread a very thin, even layer of the seed mix onto both trays. Put the seed mix in the oven to bake, setting a timer to go off after 3 hours.

4. When the timer goes off, turn the seed mixture over to help it dry. Return the trays to the oven and bake for a further 3 hours, then take them out and let the seed mixture cool completely on the trays.

5. Cut the cooked cracker sheet into squares with a knife or break it into pieces. The crackers can be stored in an airtight container at room temperature for 2–4 weeks.

Port, Peppercorn and Chicken Liver Pâté

Serves 8-10

This delicious pâté goes wonderfully with our linseed crackers, but it's also a yummy snack on its own or served with your favourite fresh veggies. It can be made and kept chilled up to four days ahead.

1 cup port

1 garlic clove, sliced

1 tablespoon rosemary leaves, plus 1 small sprig extra

16 black peppercorns

250 g butter, at room temperature

500 g chicken livers, all white sinew removed, rinsed, patted dry

4 eschalots, finely chopped

sea salt

ground white pepper

¼ cup easy chicken broth (see recipe on page 133)

1½ teaspoons powdered gelatine

1. Combine the port, garlic and rosemary in a small saucepan over a medium heat with 4 black peppercorns. (Save the rest of the peppercorns to use later.) Bring to the boil, then boil for 4–5 minutes, or until the liquid has reduced by half. Strain the liquid into a small, heat-proof bowl and set it aside.

2. Melt 1 tablespoon of the butter in a large, heavy frying pan over a medium heat. When it's foaming, cook the chicken livers, in batches, for 1 minute each side, or until golden on the outside but still pink in the middle. (You don't want to overcook the livers, as it makes the pâté grainy.) Transfer the livers to a heat-proof plate.

3. Add the eschalots to the same pan over a medium heat and cook, stirring, for 2 minutes, or until softened. Stir in half the port mixture and the cooked livers, toss together for 30 seconds and then take the pan off the heat.

4. Transfer the liver mixture to a food processor and process until smooth, scraping the side of the bowl down occasionally. Press the mixture through a sieve into a bowl, then discard any solids left in the sieve.

5. Return the liver mixture to a clean food processor bowl and add the remaining butter. Process until the butter is very well incorporated and the mixture is silky smooth, then season lightly.

TIP: It's crucial to buy very fresh, moist livers with shiny flesh. Once you get home from the butcher, unwrap the livers immediately and trim away all the white sinew. Rinse them under cold water and pat dry with paper towel. Put them on a plate, cover with cling film and keep chilled for up to 2 days before making the pâté.

6. Spoon the pâté mixture into a 4-cup capacity ceramic or glass serving dish and level the top. Cover the surface directly with cling film and chill for 1 hour.

7. Gently heat the remaining port mixture and the stock in a small saucepan over a low heat. Sprinkle the gelatine in, then whisk until it's completely dissolved and the mixture is smooth. Transfer to a heat-proof jug and let it cool for 5 minutes, then carefully pour it over the surface of the chilled pâté. Scatter the remaining peppercorns over the top and decorate with the extra sprig of rosemary. Chill for 6 hours, or overnight if time permits.

8. Take the pâté out of the fridge and let it stand at room temperature for 5 minutes. Serve the pâté with our linseed crackers (see recipe on page 125) or your favourite veggies.

Luke's Spicy Kale Chips

Serves 4

Luke says: 'Okay, so I have to admit I cannot stop eating these when I make a batch! And I trust you will be the same. What I really love is that you can flavour them in so many different ways with spices, herbs, nuts, seeds and veggies.'

50 g sunflower seeds, soaked overnight and drained

1 garlic clove, peeled

½ teaspoon dried chilli flakes (or more, if you like the heat)

2 tablespoons lemon juice

4 tablespoons coconut oil, plus extra to grease the tray

sea salt

1 bunch kale, stems removed, leaves torn into large pieces

1. Preheat your oven to 120°C, then grease a large baking tray and line it with baking paper.
2. Combine the sunflower seeds, garlic, chilli flakes, lemon juice, coconut oil and a pinch of sea salt in a food processor and blend to a coarse paste.
3. Put the paste in a large bowl, then add the kale and toss to coat it evenly.
4. Arrange the kale in a single layer on the tray and bake for 40–50 minutes, or until it's crispy. Let the chips cool and store them in an airtight container.

TIP: Kale leaves burn easily, so don't overcook them. (Much like we did in our very first episode of My Kitchen Rules.)

Raw Cashew Sour Cream

Makes 2 cups

This recipe is a wonderful alternative to your typical dairy-laden dipping sauce. Made with nutrient-rich cashews, this raw sour cream makes an awesome accompaniment to our crispy chilli chicken (see recipe on page 9) or linseed crackers (see recipe on page 125).

2 cups raw cashews, soaked for at least 8 hours, rinsed

3 tablespoons apple cider vinegar

½ teaspoon salt

juice of 1 lemon

½ cup filtered water

1. Put all the ingredients in a food processor, then process until smooth and creamy. You might have to stop and scrape the side down a couple of times.
2. Serve the cashew cream with chips or crackers, or keep it in the fridge in an airtight container for up to a week.

Garlic Aioli

Makes 2 cups

Luke says: 'I love aioli and I love garlic, so why not combine those loves and create some food-in-mouth magic? Here you go – thank me later!'

2 garlic cloves, peeled

2 egg yolks

juice of ½ lemon

sea salt

1 cup avocado oil

TIP: This aioli is wicked with our crispy skin barra – see the recipe on page 18.

1. Put the garlic cloves, egg yolks, lemon juice and a pinch of sea salt in a food processor and mix well to combine. Scrape the side down a couple of times to make sure the garlic cloves break down completely.
2. Turn the food processor back on and very slowly start to pour in the avocado oil – we really mean SUPER slow, okay? Once the mixture thickens, you'll have your aioli. If the mixture is too thick, add a little more avocado oil.

Whipped Coconut Cream

Makes 2 cups

Whipped coconut cream makes a great addition to just about any dessert. You can add any flavourings you like, such as vanilla seeds or maple syrup, or mix through chopped nuts to add some crunch to the lovely smooth texture. You'll need to plan ahead just a little – the cans of coconut cream need to go in the fridge overnight.

2 × 400 ml cans coconut cream

Optional flavourings

1 tablespoon maple syrup

1 teaspoon mixed spice

2 vanilla beans, seeds scraped

½ cup macadamias, finely chopped and toasted

½ cup flaked coconut, toasted

1. Chill the cans of coconut cream in the fridge overnight, so they'll be ready to go when you are.
2. About half an hour before you're ready to start work, put a mixing bowl in the freezer to chill.
3. When you're ready to get started, take the chilled bowl from the freezer. Open the chilled cans of coconut cream, then spoon the thick layer of cream off the top and into the chilled bowl. You will need 1½ cups of this firm cream. (You can use the leftover coconut milk in your breakfast smoothies.)
4. Using an electric mixer, whisk the chilled cream until soft peaks form. Gently fold through any additional flavourings, then keep the cream chilled until ready to serve.

TIP: Whipped Coconut Cream will keep in an airtight container in the fridge for 2–3 days.

Coconut Kefir

Serves 2

Kefir is a delicious, fizzy and refreshing drink that can help to restore your intestinal flora after you've been sick, or when you've been taking antibiotics. You can use water as a base, but we love the flavour of young coconut water. A shot of this kefir is not only great tasting but also great for you!

3 young coconuts

1 packet vegetable starter culture

1. Open the coconuts and strain the coconut water into a sterilised 750 ml jar.
2. Add the vegetable starter culture to the coconut water and use a non-metallic spoon to stir it in.
3. Cover the mouth of the jar with a piece of muslin and secure it firmly with a large elastic band. Put it in a dark spot for 24–48 hours and leave it to ferment. The kefir is ready when the water has turned cloudy white.

TIP: You can test if the kefir is ready by tasting it. After 24 hours, pour some into a glass. It should taste sour, with no sweetness left, like coconut beer. Some batches are fizzier than others, but all are beneficial. If it still tastes a little sweet, put it back in the pantry for another 24 hours.

Minty Tonic for Digestion

Serves 1

The ingredients in this simple tonic are all well known for their stomach-soothing properties. Use this drink as a gentle aid to digestion, or just as a warm drink on a cold night before you go to bed.

½ cup mint leaves

½ teaspoon fennel seeds

3 cm piece ginger, peeled, chopped

1. Using a mortar and pestle, pound all the ingredients until a coarse paste forms.
2. Transfer the paste to a heat-proof jug and pour 200 ml of boiling water over the top. Let it steep for 15 minutes, then strain the liquid into a serving glass. Drink warm.

Easy Chicken Broth

Serves 10–12

Nothing says 'winter warmer' like a hearty chicken broth. Great for soups and curries, it is also ideal as a warming drink to start your day (see recipe on page 134). You can add whatever you have in the garden or the fridge, just stay away from foods that will make your broth bitter, like broccoli, turnip, cabbage and brussels sprouts. Herbs give extra flavour and have medicinal benefits, too. Parsley, rosemary, oregano, thyme, curry leaves, kaffir lime and bay leaves are some of our absolute faves!

1–1½ whole chickens, jointed (get your butcher to do that for you!)

5 litres filtered water

2 tablespoons apple cider vinegar

2 onions, roughly chopped

2 carrots, roughly chopped

4 stalks celery, roughly chopped

2 leeks, roughly chopped

1 garlic bulb, smashed up

1 tablespoon black peppercorns, lightly crushed

2 large handfuls flat-leaf parsley

herbs of your choosing

1. Put the chicken pieces in a large saucepan and add the filtered water. Add the vinegar, onions, carrots, celery, leeks, garlic and peppercorns and bring to the boil. Add the herbs.

2. Turn the heat down to low and simmer for 6–12 hours. The longer you cook the broth, the more the flavours will develop.

3. Strain the broth through a fine sieve into a large container, then cover it and put it in the fridge to cool. Remove the congealed fat that rises to the top and reserve it for cooking, then transfer the stock to smaller, airtight containers and refrigerate or freeze until needed.

TIP: The broth can be stored in the fridge for up to 4 days or frozen for up to 3 months.

Morning Bone Broth

Serves 1

Nourishing and warming, a cup of bone broth is the perfect start to the day. It tastes good and helps to heal a damaged gut. This recipe uses chicken, but you can mix it up and use beef or fish stock. Heck, you could even make a kangaroo broth! You can always add some veggies or your protein of choice to make it more of a soup or meal.

300–400 ml chicken broth
  (see recipe on page 133)

1 teaspoon ground turmeric

pinch of ground cumin

generous squeeze of lemon juice

sea salt

1. Pour the hot broth into a large mug, then stir in the turmeric, cumin, lemon juice and a pinch of salt and give it a good stir.

Roasted Beef Bone Broth

Makes about 4½ litres

This broth is delicious served on its own as a warming drink, or use it in recipes as you would a beef stock.

2 kg meaty beef bones

sea salt and ground black pepper

2 tablespoons apple cider vinegar

2 carrots, chopped

4 stalks celery, chopped

2 brown onions, chopped

½ small bunch flat-leaf parsley, torn in half

4 dried bay leaves

10 black peppercorns

4 litres filtered water

TIP: Be sure to keep your kitchen well ventilated while cooking the broth, as the smell can be quite strong. Turn on your stove's extractor fan and open all windows and doors.

1. Preheat your oven to 220°C, then put the beef bones in a large roasting pan. Season with salt and pepper. Bake for 30 minutes, or until caramelised.

2. Transfer the roasted bones and any pan juices to a large saucepan. Add all the remaining ingredients, making sure you leave a 4 cm gap between the liquid and the top of the pan.

3. Put the pan over a high heat and bring to the boil. Turn the heat down to low and let the broth simmer gently, partially covered, for 12 hours, topping up with more filtered water as needed so that the bones are always covered.

4. Use a large slotted spoon to skim away any impurities and froth that rise to the surface as the broth simmers. Take the pan off the heat and let the broth cool to room temperature.

5. Drain the broth through a fine strainer, then pour the strained liquid into airtight containers. You can store the broth in the fridge for up to a week, or in the freezer for up to 6 months. When it is chilled, your broth will separate into a fat layer, a gelatinous layer and a liquid layer. Once reheated, the separate layers will combine again.

Morning Elixir

Serves 1

A sweet and spicy alternative to the traditional breakfast tea, this fiery little elixir will kickstart your digestion and give you a great wake-me-up to boot!

1 small garlic clove, sliced

2 teaspoons finely grated fresh turmeric

¼ teaspoon chilli powder

½ teaspoon ground cinnamon

½ teaspoon maple syrup

juice and finely grated zest of ½ large lemon

1. Put all the ingredients together in a mug and pour in 200 ml of boiling water. Let it steep for 10 minutes, then serve warm. You'll need a spoon for stirring, as the spices tend to settle on the bottom of the mug.

Beet Kvass

Makes about 4 cups

This slightly tangy and lightly bubbly drink makes a delicious digestive aid, packed with fermented goodness.

4 large beetroots, peeled and chopped

2 lemon slices

⅓ cup sea salt

filtered water

1. Put the beetroot, lemon slices and salt in a 1 litre sterilised glass jar.

2. Pour over enough filtered water to cover the beetroot mixture by at least 4 cm. Leave at least a 5 cm gap between the beetroot mixture and the rim of the jar.

3. Cover the mouth of the jar with a piece of muslin and secure it firmly with a large elastic band. Set aside in a warm spot in your kitchen (the top of the fridge is quite good) and let the beetroot ferment for 2–3 days.

4. Strain the beetroot mixture through a sieve into a second sterilised jar. The kvass should be slightly thick and bubbly. The kvass will keep stored in the fridge for up to 2 months, and should be consumed as a shot (30–40 ml).

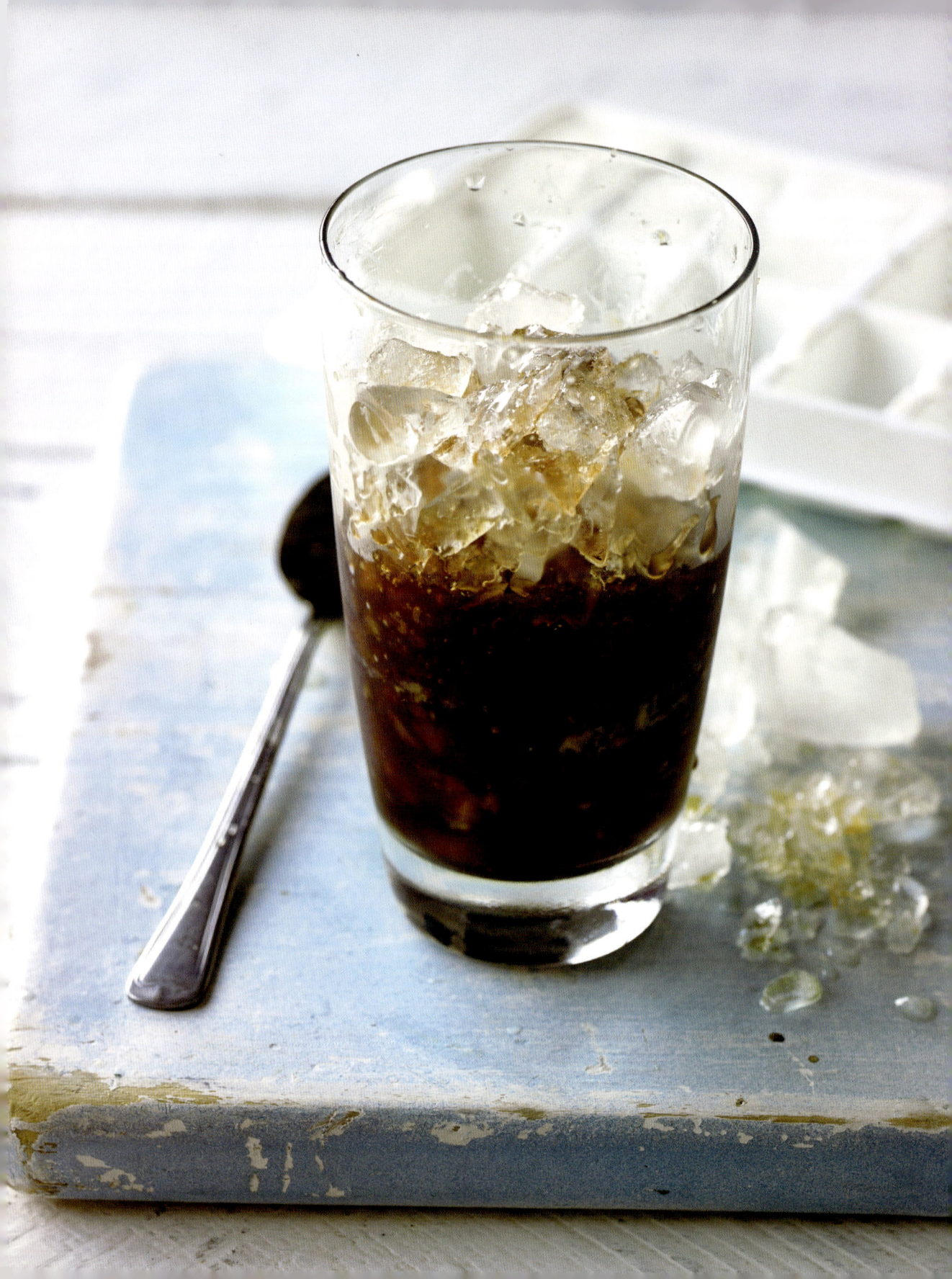

Burnt Butter Fat-Washed Iced Coffee

Serves 1

Instead of a latte or flat white, why not make this delicious clean coffee? The good fats are the perfect alternative to that takeaway cup.

⅓ cup espresso coffee

40 g butter

crushed ice and maple syrup, to serve

1. Pour the warm espresso into a heat-proof glass.
2. Melt the butter in a small frying pan over a medium-low heat and let it cook, swirling the pan occasionally, for 1–2 minutes, or until the butter starts to turn golden and smells nutty.
3. Immediately pour the hot burnt butter over the espresso in the glass. Let it stand at room temperature for 2 hours, then put it in the fridge for 2 hours, or until the fat has solidified on top of the coffee.
4. Discard the solidified fat, then fill the glass with crushed ice and spoon a small amount of maple syrup over it to taste. Serve with a tall spoon and straw.

Nut Berry Smoothie

Serves 1

When they're under stress, our bodies produce free radicals – molecules or ions with unpaired electrons that cause cellular damage. Antioxidants fight free radicals, helping to redress the balance – and this simple recipe is packed with them.

1 cup coconut milk or
  coconut water

1 cup mixed berries

1 tablespoon nut butter

1 tablespoon raw cacao powder

1. Throw all the ingredients in a blender and process until smooth.
2. Pour into a glass and serve.

Green and Orange Smoothie

Serves 2

2 oranges

large handful kale or Tuscan
  cabbage

1 avocado, halved, stone removed
  and peeled

2 teaspoons chia seeds

1 cup chopped mango, frozen

300 ml coconut milk or
  coconut water

1. Throw all the ingredients in a blender and process until smooth.
2. Pour into two glasses and serve.

TIP: If you like your smoothies thicker or thinner, add a little more or less coconut milk.

The Go-To Smoothie

Serves 2

Need more stamina in your life? Maca is a powder derived from a Peruvian root, known by locals as a potent source of energy, providing power and endurance. We use it as a training supplement, but it tastes good, too!

1½ frozen bananas

1 tablespoon tahini

handful macadamias

1 teaspoon maca

300 ml coconut milk

1 teaspoon chia seeds

1 tablespoon bee pollen (optional)

1. Throw all the ingredients, except the bee pollen, in a blender and process until smooth.
2. Pour into two glasses, sprinkle with the bee pollen (if using) for added protein and minerals, then serve.

Green Paws Smoothie

Serves 2

The taste and smell of pawpaw always takes us back to South-East Asia – a wonderful part of the world. Pawpaw is delicious and a powerful anti-inflammatory to boot!

1 frozen banana

2 bunches English spinach

1 pawpaw, seeds removed, peeled

400 ml coconut milk or
   coconut water

1. Throw all the ingredients in a blender and process until smooth.
2. Pour into two glasses and serve.

TIP: Try adding the flesh of half a young coconut to this delicious smoothie.

Beetroot and Ginger Smoothie

Serves 2

We love beets . . . packed full of goodness, they help to fight inflammation and support your immune system. You'll feel like a million dollars after this smoothie.

2 beetroots, peeled and chopped

large handful baby spinach
  or kale

2 cm piece ginger, peeled and
  roughly chopped

½ lemon, peeled and seeded

½ orange, peeled and seeded

large handful mint leaves

300 ml coconut water

1. Blend all the ingredients together and drink up!

Coconut and Kale Kickstart Smoothie

Serves 2

With these two superfoods in one smoothie, you can't go wrong!

1½ frozen bananas

2 handfuls kale

½ pineapple, peeled, or ½ mango, peeled, stone removed

½ cup young coconut flesh

1 tablespoon chia seeds

200 ml coconut milk or coconut water

1. Throw all the ingredients in a blender and process until smooth.
2. Pour into two glasses and serve.

Index

A

activated nuts and seeds 122
aioli, garlic 129
apple crumble slice 103
avocado
    guacamole 28
    lime mousse with toasted nut crumble 39
    smash 24

B

baking powder/bicarb soda ix
barramundi, crispy skin with pico de gallo
    18
beef ix
    burgers or meatballs 17
    kiwi marinated skirt steak 27
    meatloaf, mum's 67
    meatloaves, mini with avo smash 24
    roasted bone broth 135
    short ribs with cauli rice 80
beet
    and ginger smoothie 142
    kvass 137
berries
    coconut tartlets 88
    raspberry coconut truffles 104
    smoothie, nut berry 140
blini, tea-smoked trout 32
breakfast, Scott's 121
broth
    chicken, easy 133
    chicken poached in chicken broth 64
    morning bone 134
    roasted beef bone 135
burgers or meatballs 17

C

cacao
    chip cookies 99
    self-saucing pudding 100
cakes
    Christmas, individual 57
    Neapolitan ice-cream 47
    red velvet celebration 44
    Tess's spiced dream cake 111
caponata 79
    caponata-stuffed pork belly 79
cashew, raw sour cream 129
cauliflower
    cauli rice 80
    korma curry 14
chicken
    broth, easy 133
    crispy chilli 9
    noodle soup 75
    pâté, Luke and Scott's 31
    poached in chicken broth 64
chilli
    coconut dipping sauce 13
    crispy chicken 9
chocolate
    Easter eggs 108
    ice-cream 47
    raspberry coconut truffles 104
    self-saucing cacao pudding 100
    salted caramel fudge 40
    topping 40
chorizo stuffing 21
Christmas
    cakes, individual 57
    pudding with spiced cream 49–50

coconut
  and kale kickstart smoothie 143
  and mango semifreddo 43
  berry tartlets 88
  cream, whipped 130
  kefir 131
  products ix
  raspberry truffles 104
  waffles, chargrilled coconut 96
coconut oil ix
coffee ix
  iced, burnt butter fat-washed 139
cookies, cacao chip 99
cooler months
  apple crumble slice 103
  beef short ribs with cauli rice 80
  caponata-stuffed pork belly 79
  chicken, poached in chicken broth 64
  chicken noodle soup 75
  coconut berry tartlets 88
  cookies, cacao chip 99
  Easter eggs 108
  hazelnut butter cups 91
  hot cross buns 107
  jalapeños, pork-and-fennel stuffed 76
  lamb necks, braised 63
  lamb shoulder, twelve-hour-roasted 72
  lemon curd creams, chilled 92
  meatloaf, mum's 67
  pudding, self-saucing cacao 100
  pumpkin pie, sweet 95
  quail scotch eggs 84
  rabbit stroganoff 83
  raspberry coconut truffles 104
  roast pork with caraway seeds 71
  terrine, pork and pistachio 87
  Tess's spiced dream cake 111
  truffles, raspberry coconut 104

  waffles, chargrilled coconut 96
  wild mushroom soup 68
crackers, linseed 125
cream
  raw cashew sour 129
  spiced 50
  whipped coconut 130
croquettes, sweet potato and crab 13
crumb coating 13, 28
crumble 52
  apple crumble slice 103
  lime mousse with toasted nut crumble 39
curry
  cauliflower korma 14
  paste 14
custard 51

D
dates ix
desserts *see also* sweet treats
  apple crumble slice 103
  Christmas pudding with spiced cream
    49–50
  coconut and mango semifreddo 43
  coconut cream, whipped 130
  lemon curd creams, chilled 92
  lime mousse with toasted nut crumble 39
  mango lime chia pudding 36
  Neapolitan ice-cream cake 47
  pudding, self-saucing cacao 100
  pumpkin pie, sweet 95
  red velvet celebration cake 44
  trifle, summer 51–2
  waffles, chargrilled coconut 96
drinks *see also* smoothies
  beet kvass 137
  coconut kefir 131
  iced coffee, burnt butter fat-washed 139

minty tonic for digestion 132
morning elixir 136

E

Easter eggs 108
eggs ix
    Easter 108
    frittata, party 6
    quail scotch 84
elixir, morning 136

F

fennel
    jalapeños, pork-and-fennel stuffed 76
fermented veggies 117
fish ix
    barramundi, crispy skin with pico de gallo
        18
    blini, tea-smoked trout 32
    snapper, whole with fennel and pistachio
        crust 5
    tacos, crispy fish with guacamole 28
focaccia, garlic and rosemary 22
frittata, party 6
fruit ix

G

garlic
    aioli 129
    and rosemary focaccia 22
go-to smoothie, the 141
green and orange smoothie 140
green paws smoothie 141
guacamole 28

H

hazelnut butter cups 91
honey ix

hot cross buns 107

I

iced coffee, burnt butter fat-washed 139
ices and ice-cream
    chocolate ice-cream 47
    icy poles 35
    Neapolitan ice-cream cake 47
    strawberry ice-cream 47
    vanilla ice-cream 47
ingredients, notes on ix

J

jalapeños, pork-and-fennel stuffed 76
jelly 51
juices, citrus ix

K

kale
    chips, Luke's spicy 128
    coconut and, kickstart smoothie 143
    smoothie, green and orange 140
kefir, coconut 131
kiwi marinated skirt steak 27

L

lamb ix
    burgers or meatballs 17
    necks, braised 63
    shoulder, twelve-hour-roasted 72
lemon
    buttercream 44
    curd creams, chilled 92
lime mousse with toasted nut crumble
    39
linseed crackers 125

M

maca 141
mango lime chia pudding 36
maple syrup ix
meatballs 17
meatloaf
    mini with avo smash 24
    mum's 67
morning bone broth 134
mushroom, wild soup 68

N

nuoc cham 10
nuts
    and seeds, activated 122
    hazelnut butter cups 91
    raw cashew sour cream 129
    smoothie, nut berry 140

O

olive oil ix

P

panforte, festive 54
pâté
    Luke and Scott's 31
    port, peppercorn and chicken liver 126
pepper, black ix
pico de gallo 18
pie
    crust 95
    sweet pumpkin 95
pork ix
    caponata-stuffed belly 79
    jalapeños, pork-and-fennel stuffed 76
    roast with caraway seeds 71
    terrine, pistachio and 87
port, peppercorn and chicken liver pâté 126

prawn salad with nuoc cham 10
pudding
    Christmas with spiced cream 49–50
    mango lime chia 36
    self-saucing cacao 100
pumpkin
    filling 95
    pie, sweet 95

Q

quail scotch eggs 84

R

rabbit stroganoff 83
raspberry coconut truffles 104

S

salad, prawn with nuoc cham 10
salsa, pico de gallo 18
salted caramel choc fudge 40
sauces
    chilli coconut dipping 13
    nuoc cham 10
sauerkraut 118
sea salt ix
seafood
    barramundi, crispy skin with pico de gallo 18
    blini, tea-smoked trout 32
    croquettes, sweet potato and crab 13
    prawn salad with nuoc cham 10
    snapper, whole with fennel and pistachio crust 5
    tacos, crispy fish with guacamole 28
semifreddo, coconut and mango 43
smoothies
    beetroot and ginger 142
    coconut and kale kickstart 143

go-to, the 141
green and orange 140
green paws 141
nut berry 140
snapper, whole with fennel and pistachio
crust 5
soup
chicken broth, easy 133
chicken noodle 75
morning bone broth 134
roasted beef bone broth 135
wild mushroom 68
spiced cream 50
strawberry ice-cream 47
stroganoff, rabbit 83
stuffing, chorizo 21
sweet potato
croquettes, crab and 13
sweet treats *see also* desserts
apple crumble slice 103
cookies, cacao chip 99
Easter eggs 108
hazelnut butter cups 91
hot cross buns 107
icy poles 35
panforte, festive 54
salted caramel choc fudge 40
Tess's spiced dream cake 111
waffles, chargrilled coconut 96

T

tacos, crispy fish with guacamole 28
tartlets, coconut berry 88
tea ix
terrine, pork and pistachio 87
tonic, minty for digestion 132
trifle, summer 51–2
truffles, raspberry coconut 104

turkey, Christmas with chorizo stuffing 21

V

vanilla ice-cream 47
vegetables ix
fermented 117
kale chips, Luke's spicy 128
sauerkraut 118
vinegar
apple cider ix

W

waffles, chargrilled coconut 96
warmer months
barramundi, crispy skin with pico de gallo
18
blini, tea-smoked trout 32
burgers or meatballs 17
cauliflower korma curry 14
Christmas cakes, individual 57
Christmas pudding with spiced cream
49–50
coconut and mango semifreddo 43
crispy chilli chicken 9
croquettes, sweet potato and crab 13
focaccia, garlic and rosemary 22
frittata, party 6
icy poles 35
kiwi marinated skirt steak 27
lime mousse with toasted nut crumble 39
mango lime chia pudding 36
meatloaves, mini with avo smash 24
Neapolitan ice-cream cake 47
panforte, festive 54
pâté, Luke and Scott's 31
prawn salad with nuoc cham 10
red velvet celebration cake 44
salted caramel choc fudge 40

snapper, whole with fennel and pistachio
crust 5
tacos, crispy fish with guacamole 28
trifle, summer 51–2
turkey, Christmas with chorizo stuffing 21

Y
year-round essentials
aioli, garlic 129
beet kvass 137
chicken broth, easy 133
coconut cream, whipped 130
coconut kefir 131
iced coffee, burnt butter fat-washed 139
kale chips, Luke's spicy 128
linseed crackers 125
minty tonic for digestion 132
morning bone broth 134
morning elixir 136
nuts and seeds, activated 122
pâté, port, peppercorn and chicken liver
126
raw cashew sour cream 129
roasted beef bone broth 135
sauerkraut 118
Scott's breakfast 121
veggies, fermented 117

GET IN TOUCH WITH LUKE:

www.lukehines.com

Tweet me:
@LukeHinesOnline

Instagram me:
@LukeHinesOnline

Facebook me:
www.facebook.com/lukehinesonline

GET IN TOUCH WITH SCOTT:

www.scottgoodingproject.com

Tweet me:
@ScottyFit

Instagram me:
@ScottyFit

Facebook me:
www.facebook.com/scottgoodingfitness